The Ultimate Medical Student Guide to Dermatology

Nicholas Brownstone

The Ultimate Medical Student Guide to Dermatology

Springer

Nicholas Brownstone, MD
The Kimberly and Eric J. Waldman
Department of Dermatology
Icahn School of Medicine at Mount Sinai
New York, NY, USA

ISBN 978-3-031-98764-9 ISBN 978-3-031-98765-6 (eBook)
https://doi.org/10.1007/978-3-031-98765-6

This Springer imprint is published by the registered company Springer Nature Switzerland AG
The registered company address is: Gewerbestrasse 11, 6330 Cham, Switzerland

To my parents, Judy and Doug, and my sisters, Nina and Julie—thank you for instilling in me the importance and true meaning of family. You have always been there for me to celebrate the good times in life and help me through the hard times and for that I am forever grateful.

To my cousins Randy, Chris, Glenn, Nicole, and Ryan—thank you for showing me what it means to be successful both personally and professionally.

To Nanny, Pop, and Aunt Marie and for everyone else who is not with us anymore, but is with us in Spirit.

To every patient who has trusted me with their care.

Foreword by Sandra Lee

Dermatology is often seen as a specialized and disparate field, yet its relevance spans across nearly every discipline of medicine. Whether diagnosing a life-threatening rash in the emergency room, recognizing a cutaneous manifestation of systemic disease, or simply managing common conditions like acne and eczema in primary care, every physician—regardless of specialty—must have a solid foundation in dermatology.

Despite this, dermatology remains one of the most underemphasized subjects in medical education. Many students receive limited exposure during their training, leaving them unprepared for both board exams and real-world clinical encounters. Yet, skin disorders account for a significant proportion of primary care visits, and many high-yield dermatologic conditions frequently appear on standardized exams. A strong grasp of dermatology is not just beneficial—it is essential for success in both medical school and clinical practice.

That is precisely why *The Ultimate Medical Student Guide to Dermatology* is such a valuable resource. This book condenses the immense field of dermatology into a concise, high-yield reference tailored specifically for medical students. Designed for both board review and clinical practice, it presents key concepts in an accessible format, ensuring that students can quickly and confidently recognize, diagnose, and manage important dermatologic conditions.

What sets this guide apart is its clarity, practicality, and clinical relevance. It goes beyond rote memorization, helping students develop a true understanding of dermatologic principles that will serve them not only on exams but throughout their medical careers. Whether you are preparing for Step 1, Step 2, or your clinical rotations, this book will be your go-to reference—one that bridges the gap between classroom knowledge and patient care.

Mastering dermatology is not just about passing exams; it's about becoming a more competent, well-rounded physician. With this guide in your hands, you will hopefully be equipped with the knowledge and confidence to recognize and manage skin conditions more effectively, ensuring better outcomes for your future patients.

This book has the potential to become the definitive dermatology resource for medical students, and I have no doubt that it will.

Welcome to *The Ultimate Medical Student Guide to Dermatology*—your essential companion for board exam success and clinical excellence.

Upland, CA, USA Sandra Lee, MD, FAAD "Dr. Pimple Popper"

Foreword by Terrence A. Cronin Jr.

As a dermatologist dedicated to staying passionate about dermatology, I am thrilled to recommend *The Ultimate Medical Student Guide to Dermatology*, authored by Nicholas Brownstone, MD, who was the chief dermatology resident at Temple University Hospital and is the host of the Cutaneous Miscellaneous: The Dermatology Residents Podcast.

In this meticulously crafted guide, Dr. Brownstone seamlessly integrates a wealth of knowledge from renowned resources like Bolognia and his own extensive clinical experience to create an unparalleled resource for medical students. Dermatology is a crucial aspect of medical practice, and this book serves as an invaluable tool for both clinical learning and board exam preparation. Dr. Brownstone's dedication to advancing the field through his research, publications, and educational endeavors shines through in this comprehensive guide. I have no doubt that this book will become the go-to quick reference for students seeking to learn and master the complexities of dermatology.

Former President American
Academy of Dermatology 2023–2024
Melbourne, FL, USA

Terrence A. Cronin Jr., MD, FAAD

Preface

I love dermatology, and I love practicing dermatology! However, I did not realize this passion until many years after graduating medical school. I began my career as a plastic and reconstructive surgery resident, completing over 3 years of surgical training. I liked plastic surgery, but something was missing for me. It was not until my first formal rotation in dermatology as an intern in plastic surgery that I realized what exactly was missing and what I truly desired as a doctor. I loved performing procedures and working with my hands, but I missed the "medical" aspects of practicing medicine. After realizing that dermatology is the perfect mix of medicine and surgery, I made the difficult decision to switch specialties in 2019 and pursue dermatology. The rest is history. Not a moment goes by that I regret my change, and it is one of the best decisions I have made in my life so far. I am so thankful that I am now in a career where I love going to work every day.

I think an issue for me, and frankly an issue for every medical student, is the limited exposure to didactic and clinical dermatology during medical school. Most medical schools only offer an hour or two on skin disease during the entirety of the 4-year medical school curriculum, with no required rotations in a dermatology clinic. This is an issue for two reasons. One reason is that many medical students who are meant to be dermatologists and would excel in the field simply choose another specialty because they are not exposed to it. The second reason is that many medical students who graduate medical school have little to no knowledge on handling even basic dermatological issues.

This book seeks to address both issues by introducing students to a career in dermatology and provides detailed and important clinical information that medical students need to know as an aspiring dermatologist or as a future physician pursuing a different specialty. Skin problems impact nearly every other medical specialty, and I am sure we all can relate to being asked by a stranger or loved one to "take a look at this spot." Furthermore, passing board exams is required by all students, and this resource also highlights high-yield board review tips presented in an easy-to-read format. This book is also perfect for physician assistant students, nurse practitioner students, and even residents in dermatology, internal medicine, family medicine, and emergency medicine.

Dermatology is more than diagnosing rashes or prescribing topical therapies; it is a window into systemic health and a specialty that requires a comprehensive approach. As you navigate the pages of this book, I encourage you to focus not just on memorizing facts but on understanding the clinical reasoning that underpins each condition.

I hope this resource serves as a stepping-stone in your journey through dermatology, helping you to develop both the knowledge and the clinical acumen required to excel in this field. Whether you're just beginning to explore dermatology, preparing for exams, or seeking to better understand skin disease as a non-dermatologist, may this book inspire confidence, curiosity, and a deeper appreciation for the complexity of skin diseases

If the knowledge gained from reading this book helps even just one patient, I view that as a success!

New York, NY, USA Nicholas Brownstone, MD

Acknowledgments

Thank you to the amazing staff at Springer Nature for helping me put this book together.

I would also like to thank my residency chair and program director, Sylvia Hsu, MD, for teaching me and inspiring me to become the best dermatologist that I can be, and Saira Agarwala, MD, for reviewing portions of this book. I would also like to acknowledge Sylvia Hsu, MD and Jayci Rhein, MD for their photo contributions.

Disclaimer

The information contained in this book is not to be substituted for clinical judgment. The author is not responsible for treatment decisions or outcomes based on the information in this book. To the fullest extent of the law, no responsibility is assumed by Springer, authors, editors, or contributors for any injury and/or damage to persons or property as a matter of products liability, negligence or otherwise, or from any use or operation of any methods, products, instructions, or ideas contained in the material herein.

Contents

Chapter 1
A Career in Dermatology

Introduction

Dermatology is an extremely unique specialty within the house of medicine. Cardiologists treat diseases of the heart but must rely on a stethoscope to exam it. Hepatobiliary surgeons must spend significant time and effort dissecting through skin, subcutaneous tissue, fascia, and muscle to address the issue they are tasked with. Psychiatrists must spend some time interviewing their patient before solidifying a diagnosis and treatment plan. Radiologists are the "eyes of medicine" but never directly see their specimen. Instead, they must rely on X-rays, CT scans, ultrasound, MRIs, and nuclear medicine to study their structure of interest.

Only the dermatologist can walk into an exam room and in some cases make a correct diagnosis in nearly 2 seconds flat! However, it takes years of intensive training to perform this feat, and diagnosing skin disease is not always this easy. Many cases require substantiative critical thinking, skin biopsies, and laboratory testing to arrive at a diagnosis and appropriate treatment regimen. However, the fact that the skin is so accessible, easily studied, and sampled makes dermatology an incredibly exciting and attractive field!

Dermatology comes from the Greek word *dermatos,* meaning skin. Human skin has over 300 million cells, covers an average area of 18.5 ft^2, and is the largest organ in the body. If you ask most people what kind of doctor a dermatologist is, they will likely say, "a skin doctor." While this is obviously true, dermatologists are also specialists in the diagnosis and management of diseases of the hair, nails, and mucous membranes. According to the American Academy of Dermatology (AAD), a board-certified dermatologist learns how to accurately diagnose and treat more than 3,000 diseases of the skin, hair, and nails (as well as cosmetic concerns) during residency.

The AAD conducted a study examining the impact of skin disease on the US population in 2016, called the Burden of Skin Disease, and discovered some incredible statistics about the field of dermatology, which included the following: (1) one

N. Brownstone, *The Ultimate Medical Student Guide to Dermatology*,
https://doi.org/10.1007/978-3-031-98765-6_1

in four Americans were impacted by skin disease; (2) skin disease cost the US Healthcare system $75 billion; and (3) one in three Americans were seen by a dermatologist. This is not surprising as dermatologists treat patients from 0 years old to greater than 100 years old and care for patients from every race, gender, and skin tone.

The Practice of Dermatology

Dermatologists manage a variety of pathologies, including autoimmune, infectious (including viral, bacterial, fungal, protozoal, worms, and infestations), malignant, inflammatory, environmental, occupational, allergic, traumatic, psychiatric, idiopathic, congenital, and iatrogenic. They examine the body from the top of the scalp to the tips of the toes (including all the folds in between). They practice medicine, surgery, pediatrics, pathology, and cosmetics. They use lasers, injectables, neurotoxins, chemical peels, liposuction, hair transplantation, sclerotherapy, phototherapy, topical medications, cosmeceuticals, over-the-counter medications/products, pills, infusions, biologics, and intralesional therapy to treat disease and enhance the skin.

They take referrals from, and consult with, nearly all other medical specialties, including surgeons and surgical subspecialties (i.e., plastic, transplant, burn), medicine and medicine subspecialties (i.e., endocrine, hematology, infectious disease, pulmonary, gastroenterology), pathologists, orthopedists, pediatricians, geriatricians, critical care/ICU physicians, rheumatologists, oncologists, ER doctors, OB/GYNs, ophthalmologists, and psychiatrists. Given this, the dermatologist can be considered the “doctor’s doctor” and the “last of the true general practitioners.”

They handle life-threating conditions such as melanoma, Stevens-Johnson Syndrome/Toxic Epidermal Necrolysis (SJS/TEN), and pemphigus vulgaris but mostly encounter diseases that are not deadly, but are life-ruining and greatly impact a patient’s quality of life. A few prominent examples of these diseases include acne, atopic dermatitis, hidradenitis suppurativa, alopecia areata, vitiligo, and psoriasis. Thus, while other doctors may save a life, the dermatologist makes it worth living.

Dermatologists typically practice in a fast-paced outpatient clinic making diagnoses, seeing follow-up patients, and performing procedures. It is difficult to describe a “typical day” for a dermatologist but one might look like the following:

- Treating nodular acne with isotretinoin.
- Making a new diagnosis of psoriasis.
- Treating severe atopic dermatitis with a biologic.
- Diagnosing and treating herpes zoster.
- Counseling a patient on granuloma annulare.
- Diagnosing the reason for a patient’s hair loss.
- Doing a total body exam for skin cancer.
- Counseling a patient on the reason for their allergic contact dermatitis.

- Performing corticosteroid injections for alopecia areata.
- Performing a shave biopsy for a suspected basal cell carcinoma.
- Making a new diagnosis of vitiligo.
- Providing reassurance to a worried patient on the benign nature of pityriasis rosea.
- Performing cryosurgery for warts.
- Treating seborrheic dermatitis.
- Performing an incision and drainage of a skin abscess.

The field is a very procedural and hands-on specialty. Dermatologists are almost always spraying, injecting, destroying skin lesions, or performing biopsies and surgical excisions during any given clinic session. Pediatric dermatology clinic may not be as procedural while Mohs surgery and cosmetic dermatology are nearly 100% procedural. A dermatologist who covers consults may be called into the hospital to diagnose or rule out a dangerous drug rash during their lunch break or after clinic as well.

Beyond an outpatient clinic, dermatologists also practice in almost every setting imaginable in the field of medicine. They see admitted patients in the hospital and patients in the intensive care units as consults. They respond to the Emergency Room when necessary for consultations as well. Dermatologists can also see patients virtually through telehealth, which has become a more popular venue since the COVID-19 pandemic. Some dermatologists even perform laser procedures or surgical procedures in the Operating Room.

Dermatologists can also serve in many leadership roles throughout hospitals and health systems. In fact, a former president of the American Medical Association (the largest physician organization in the world) is a dermatologist. Furthermore, a dermatologist is currently serving as a US Congressman. Outside of practicing medicine, dermatologists can consult with skincare companies or pharmaceutical companies on the newest dermatology medications and skincare products. Dermatologists are critical in helping to design and perform clinical trials that allow new medications to be FDA approved for patients. They are also critical in ensuring that over-the-counter skincare products are safe, effective, and desirable for consumers.

The practice of dermatology is rooted in a technical language. There are words and terms that are rarely used in other fields of medicine. A technical language is extremely important when accurately describing skin lesions and skin rashes so another dermatologist who might consult on the case or see the patient for follow up can more accurately diagnose and treat the patient. These specific and technical terms help paint a very narrow and focused picture and can more efficiently indicate the correct diagnosis. Listed below are increasing more specific descriptions of a skin lesion. One can see how the technical language of dermatology helps paint a precise picture of the correct diagnosis, while vague language is not helpful.

- A lesion.
- A raised lesion.
- A raised reddish/purplish lesion.

- A violaceous papule.
- A violaceous, polygonal, papule.
- A violaceous, polygonal, papule that is pruritic.
- A violaceous, polygonal, flat-topped, pruritic, papule with Wickham's striae.
- A violaceous, polygonal, flat-topped, pruritic, papule with Wickham's striae on the flexor wrist.

The language of dermatology takes years to master. Many medical schools only offer an hour or two of dermatology lectures throughout the entirety of the 4-year curriculum with no official clinical rotations on a dermatology service or in a dermatology clinic. Thus, many dermatology residents feel like they are "starting medical school all over again" in residency due to the very limited clinical and didactic exposure to the specialty as a medical student. There are numerous confusing terms, similar sounding names, buzzwords/phrases, misnomers, and eponyms that make learning dermatology challenging. Parts II and IV of this book help address this issue for students learning dermatology. Furthermore, actively seeking rotations/electives in a dermatology clinic and finding a mentor in the field will also help.

Matching into Dermatology

Dermatology is an incredibly competitive specialty! The website "Med School Insiders" (https://medschoolinsiders.com) performed an analysis of 22 medical specialties with the 2024 National Residency Matching Program (NRMP) Charting Outcomes™ data and assessed six factors, including average match rate, Step 1 score (even though Step 1 changed to pass/fail in 2022, the students included in the 2024 data took Step 1 when it was still scored), Step 2 CK score, number of publications, percentage of matriculants that were AOA, and percentage of applicants from a top 40 NIH-funded medical school. Based on this analysis, the authors found that dermatology was the #1 most competitive specialty ahead of neurosurgery, plastic surgery, orthopedic surgery, and otorhinolaryngology.

Given this, many medical students are choosing to take a research year in medical school dedicated to dermatology. This goal of this research year is to conduct research and gain the support of a nationally recognized dermatologist who can support and advocate for the applicant during the residency application and interview process. An added benefit of a research year at a different institution is exposure to another dermatology department. If the medical student works hard and makes a positive impression, then they might have a higher chance of matching at a competitive program, where they may not have been known before. The same holds true for audition/away rotations.

While a research year is very popular option, they are by no means necessary to match into dermatology, and the advantages and disadvantages should be discussed with trusted advisors and mentors. Performance on away/audition rotations is also one of the most important factors in matching into dermatology. Unfortunately, a medical student can only complete a few of these rotations. Medical students should not be too worried or focused on getting the right diagnosis on these rotations (they are students after all) but should focus on being a team player, fitting in with the other residents and not being too overeager or too much of an annoyance. The best piece of advice is to demonstrate passion and a true interest in the field of dermatology. Diagnoses that were seen in clinic that day should be studied and reviewed that same night. If any research projects become available during that rotation, the student should be eager to help out and learn about that topic more in-depth.

A strong and genuine letter from a nationally recognized dermatologist and a phone call or e-mail from that person to other programs during the residency application process is an important factor in successfully obtaining a residency spot in dermatology. Other key attributes of successful applicants include having a competitive USMLE Step 2 score and being well-liked and fitting in with the department during audition/away rotations. Many applicants who match at specific programs were well liked by that program, fit with the culture of the program and the personalities of the residents, hustled and worked hard during their rotation, did not complain, and showed a sincere interest in learning dermatology. The medical students who become the best dermatology residents and the best dermatologists are the ones that work the hardest and are passionate about practicing dermatology and getting better throughout their entire career.

The requirement to become a board-certified dermatologist after medical school requires a “1 + 3” model of training. This means 1 year of internship is needed along with 3 years of dermatology residency. The internship year is usually taken in medicine or surgery, but a broad-based internship experience (such as a transitional year) may be accepted by the American Board of Dermatology. The internship year does not have to be completed at the same hospital as the dermatology residency, and many residents may choose to experience a different city or hospital for a year before moving somewhere else for 3 or more years of training. As such, medical students applying to dermatology must apply to and interview at both dermatology residency programs and separate 1-year internship programs during their interview season.

Dermatology Residency

Dermatology residency is a busy and exciting time! While it may not be as intensive as a surgical residency or hospital-based residency, it is by no means “easier,” just different. While some non-dermatology residents may spend more time in the hospital, the amount of reading in dermatology residency makes the hours worked comparable to most other residency programs, even though the dermatology residents’ time may be spent studying at home or at the library. Dermatology residents must pass five exams to become board-certified, which includes four separate CORE exams in medical dermatology, pediatric dermatology, surgical/cosmetic dermatology, and dermatopathology, which are taken in the second and third years of residency. They most also pass the APPLIED exam, which assesses the ability to apply knowledge in clinical scenarios at the level of an independent practicing dermatologist. The APPLIED exam is taken shortly after graduating. Other expected activities during dermatology residency include giving didactic lectures, delivering grand rounds, teaching medical students/physician assistants, conducting research, performing a quality improvement project, and attending the annual American Academy of Dermatology meeting.

At its core, dermatology is a visible field, and many hours are spent studying "Kodachromes" (which is the brand name for a color reversal film introduced by the Eastman Kodak company in 1935). Before computers, dermatologists studied and reviewed cases using physical Kodachrome slides. Today, a Kodachrome is simply another word for a picture of skin disease. A lot of time is spent in residency looking at Kodachromes to learn how to recognize certain conditions in clinical practice. One of the difficulties in the practice of dermatology is that the textbook picture or Kodachrome review set may only show a handful of examples of a certain skin condition. However, in clinical practice it may manifest in many different forms or atypical presentations. Thus, an expert dermatologist knows how to recognize the many uncommon presentations of a common condition, rather than misdiagnosing the patient with a rare condition.

An uncommon presentation of a common condition may be one of many reasons why a dermatologist chooses to perform a skin biopsy. An important concept in the practice of dermatology is performing a "clinicopathologic correlation" (CPC). A CPC is the process of combining clinical information with pathological findings to help arrive at the correct diagnosis. Many medical students think the biopsy is the "answer key" but this is not the case. Just like a dermatologist who looks at a rash on the skin and studies the morphology and distribution to arrive at their best diagnosis, the dermatopathologist studies the type of cells and pattern of cells under their microscope to also arrive at their best diagnosis. However, many clinical diagnoses may fit one histological pattern and a specific histological pattern may fit many clinical diagnoses.

Many dermatology residents find learning dermatopathology difficult during residency but it is the foundation of dermatology. The dermatologist needs to have a sound and fundamental working knowledge of dermatopathology to be able to diagnosis cases that are not classic or provide more information when they are not confident about their diagnosis based solely on clinical exam. For example, a dermatologist may biopsy a psoriasiform rash on the upper trunk and get back "vacuolar interface" on the pathology report. The dermatologist must then perform a CPC and realize that subacute cutaneous lupus erythematosus (SCLE) may look like psoriasis on the skin but under the microscope appears as a vacuolar interface pattern. Thus, the diagnosis is SCLE and not psoriasis.

Dermatology Fellowships

There are numerous fellowships available to a dermatology resident after residency. Three fellowships are officially recognized as dermatology subspecialities by the American Board of Medical Specialties (ABMS) and include dermatopathology, pediatric dermatology and micrographic surgery and dermatologic oncology (commonly known as Mohs surgery fellowship). A pediatric dermatologist specializes in treating children (newborns to adolescents) with a condition that affects their skin, hair, or nails and usually sees severe pediatric skin disease, newborn rashes, challenging/complicated birthmarks, and rare genetic skin diseases. A dermatopathologist practices both dermatology and pathology and is trained to examine tissue removed during a skin biopsy with a microscope and provide a diagnosis or histological features in a report called a biopsy report or dermatopathology report. Sometimes, a dermatopathologist uses special stains or immunostains to help arrive at the correct diagnosis. Board certification in dermatopathology can also be obtained after completing a general pathology residency.

Micrographic dermatologic surgery or Mohs surgery is a special type of skin cancer surgeon who takes serial layers of very small pieces of skin, then immediately examines the tissue under a microscope. This allows the surgeon to see when the cancer stops and preserve tissue with the goal of not taking more tissue than is needed to completely remove the cancer. Mohs surgeons are also trained in reconstructive surgery to repair the defect created by removal of the tumor with plastic surgery techniques such as flaps and grafts. Mohs surgery was pioneered by and named after an American surgeon, Frederic Edward Mohs. A certifying exam is taken after completion of these fellowships and the duration is each 1 year in length. Some select fellowships may be 2 years in length with the addition of 1 year for research.

There are other dermatology fellowships available to a dermatology resident after completion of training that are not officially recognized by the ABMS but are still popular options. These fellowships include cosmetic dermatology, complex medical dermatology, and advanced surgical dermatology. Cosmetic dermatology includes further training in lasers, fillers, neurotoxins, hair restoration, liposuction, and chemical peels. Complex medical dermatology includes further training in medical dermatology patients with multiple comorbidities, medical dermatology patients who have failed multiple therapies, in-patient dermatology consults, and rare or difficult to treat dermatologic conditions. They also specialize in skin conditions that are the result of an internal medicine disease, systemic disease or autoimmune disease. A few advanced surgical dermatology fellowships even offer training in procedures like blepharoplasty and facelifts. A certifying exam is not taken after completion of these fellowships, and the duration is usually 1 year in length. There are many other niche areas of the field where dermatologists can become experts without the need to complete a fellowship. Examples of these areas include supportive oncodermatology, psychodermatology, trichology (hair diseases) and nail diseases.

The Future of Dermatology

Dermatology has always been, and will always remain, a "media darling" as it is an extremely popular topic among the mass media and on social media. Not only do we have "influencers" on social media, but we also now have "skinfluencers" who provide advice on dermatology and skin care, even without any medical training or medical degree. Misinformation is a growing threat to the field of dermatology in the current landscape of social media. Dermatologists must continue to play a critical role in combating misinformation related to skin health by actively identifying and refuting inaccurate information circulating online, educating patients on evidence-based practices, and utilizing their platform and training to disseminate reliable information through social media.

The future of dermatology is incredibly bright! It will always remain as a specialty that is important in the house of medicine. This is especially evident when a dermatologist catches an internal malignancy or systemic disease from its skin manifestations. While there has been great innovation in dermatology with the recent approval of new biologics, JAK inhibitors and topical medications for numerous skin diseases, there are still some skin diseases with no FDA-approved therapies. There are also many skin diseases that have current FDA-approved medications, but these medications are of limited efficacy.

Conclusion

Many other doctors think dermatology is easy, but this is far from the truth. It is an intellectually challenging and technically oriented specialty that takes years of training and studying to practice proficiently. Medical students who are seeking a fast-paced, intellectual, and procedure-based specialty with a ton of variety should consider dermatology as a career choice. A great place to start is by reading this book!

Chapter 2
Basic Dermatologic Terminology

Primary Lesions

Primary skin lesions represent natural skin changes that have not been altered by trauma, manipulation, treatment, or natural regression. They are the most characteristic or native appearance of skin disease.

- Macule
  - A flat discoloration that lacks surface elevation or depression (< 1 cm).
    - Examples include vitiligo or a freckle.
  - The **l** in macu**l**e can help you remember that the lesion is completely flat.
- Papule
  - A small, elevated lesion that you can feel (< 1 cm).
    - Examples include molluscum contagiosum.
  - A **pa**pule can be **palpa**ted and "pops" out of the skin.
- Patch
  - A flat discoloration that is larger than a macule (> 1 cm).
    - Examples include port wine stain and melasma.
  - Think about repairing an old pair of ripped jeans with a patch, the end result is completely flat.
- Plaque
  - An elevated, solid lesion that is larger than a papule that commonly has scale or surface change (> 1 cm).

N. Brownstone, *The Ultimate Medical Student Guide to Dermatology*,
https://doi.org/10.1007/978-3-031-98765-6_2

    - Examples include psoriasis and lichen simplex chronicus.
  - Imagine winning an award and being presented with a thick, solid gold plaque. The plaque is raised and you can feel it.
- Nodule
  - An elevated larger solid lesion that commonly lacks surface change (> 1 cm).
    - Examples include lipoma, rheumatoid nodule, and erythema nodosum.
      - You should "**nod**" and greet a **nod**ule because of how big and prominent it appears; it's a sign of respect!
- Wheal
  - An elevated, edematous firm plaque that is transitory, typically without surface change and exhibiting central pallor.
    - Examples include urticaria or dermatographism.
  - Imagine a tire/wheel on a car that is filled with air, a wheal in dermatology is caused by dermal edema and filled with fluid from leaky blood vessels.
- Vesicle
  - A small papule that contains clear fluid (< 1 cm).
    - Examples include herpes simplex, varicella, dyshidrotic eczema, and dermatitis herpetiformis.
  - Don't in**V**est in a **V**esicle because they are small and don't contain much fluid.
- Bullae
  - A larger localized fluid collection that can be filled with clear, serous, or hemorrhagic fluid (> 1 cm).
    - Examples include bullous pemphigoid, thermal burns, edema blisters, and toxic epidermal necrolysis (TEN).
  - Bullae are like bullies, they are large and scary looking!
- Pustule
  - A papule that contains purulent, cloudy material.
    - Examples include pustular psoriasis, AGEP, and acne.
  - A **P**ustule contains **P**us and can be **P**inpoint.
- Cyst
  - A specific type of nodule that contains fluid or semisolid material, a visible punctum may be appreciated.
    - Examples include infundibular cyst and pilar cyst.

  - When dealing with a **cyst**, it is usually a good idea to get an **"assist"** from someone because you will likely be expressing material from it (such as keratin).

Secondary Features

Secondary skin lesions are created by exogenous factors such scratching, rubbing, or infection. These changes may also develop as skin/skin disease changes evolve over time. Skin biopsies should be avoided on lesions with significant secondary changes as a general rule.

- Crust
  - A superficial collection of cellular debris, dried serum, blood, or pus on the surface of skin lesions.
    - Examples include impetigo and allergic contact dermatitis.
    - Also known as a scab.
  - Imagine a crusty old piece of bread, the crust is on the surface of the bread, and is easily flaked off.
- Scale
  - Hyperkeratosis or thickened stratum corneum that is due to hyperproliferation of skin cells or delayed shedding of skin cells.
    - Examples include psoriasis and actinic keratosis.
  - Imagine the plate-like scales of a dragon, they are thick and protective.
- Fissure
  - Linear cleft in the skin due to a vertical loss in epidermis and partial dermis with sharp demarcation.
    - Examples include hand eczema and atopic dermatitis.
    - Also known as a crack.
  - Imagine a large earthquake causing a fissure or crack in the ground.
- Excoriation
  - Partial loss of the epidermis usually in a linear or punctate configuration.
    - Seen in pruritic conditions such as scabies or atopic dermatitis.
    - This is a linear erosion caused by scratching.
  - The **X** in e**X**coriations looks like two scratch marks that are at angles to one another.

- Erosion
  - Partial loss of epidermis.
    - Seen in impetigo and pemphigus foliaceus.
    - Heals without scarring.
  - Beach erosion is the gradual wearing away of the sand, rocks, and soil that make up a beach. Imagine the skin surface being slowly eroded away where just a thin layer is missing.
- Ulceration
  - Full-thickness loss of epidermis that may even involve into full-thickness loss of the entire dermis or even subcutis.
    - Seen in venous stasis ulcer, decubitus ulcer, and pyoderma gangrenosum.
    - Heals with a scar.
  - The **U** in **U**lcer represents a deeper loss of the skin because it looks like a large crater.
- Atrophy
  - Thinning of the epidermis that leads to a wrinkling and shiny appearance that may include telangiectasias or stretch marks.
    - Seen in lichen sclerosus.
  - A**T**rophy causes tissue **T**hinning.
- Infarct
  - Ischemia and death of tissue that appears gray to purple to black.
    - Seen in vascular compromises like calciphylaxis or thrombosis.
  - Think about a myocardial infarction (heart attack) causing death of the heart muscle.
- Lichenification
  - A focal area of thickened skin produced by chronic scratching or rubbing with accentuated and prominent skin lines.
    - Seen in lichen simplex chronicus.
  - **LI**chenification leads to prominent **LI**nes on the skin from rubbing and scratching.

Chapter 3
The Diseases

1. Acanthosis nigricans

   - Morphology/clinical features

     – Velvety hyperpigmented plaques.
     – Onset of condition is insidious.

       - Patients are usually overweight.

     – Asymptomatic.

   - Distribution

     – Intertriginous areas and less often extensor surfaces.
     – Most frequently affected sites are the neck and axilla.

   - Etiology/pathogenesis

     – Exact pathogenesis unknown but likely related to circulating molecules that stimulate epidermal proliferation.
     – Can also be a paraneoplastic condition.
     – In rare cases, drug triggers include OCPs, protease inhibitors, niacin, and human growth hormone.

   - Internal sequelae/comorbidities

     – Associated with insulin resistance and diabetes mellitus.
     – Paraneoplastic acanthosis nigricans is characterized by rapid onset of disease in multiple flexural areas.

       - Associated with adenocarcinomas (stomach, GI, and GU).
       - 25% of patients also have tripe palms.

N. Brownstone, *The Ultimate Medical Student Guide to Dermatology*,
https://doi.org/10.1007/978-3-031-98765-6_3

- Laboratory testing
  - Fasting blood glucose.
  - Hemoglobin A1C (HbA1c).
- Treatments/prognosis
  - Very hard to treat! Must counsel patients on the difficult nature of treating this condition.
  - Treat underlying disorder.
    - **Weight loss**, control of diabetes, and control of any other underlying endocrinopathy.
  - Some dermatologists may try tretinoin and ammonium lactate but these will not work very well.
- USMLE Board Review Pearls
  - Look for velvety dark plaques in the neck and axilla.
  - Associated with DM (insulin resistance), Cushing disease, polycystic ovarian syndrome (PCOS), and obesity.
  - May be a sign of underlying adenocarcinoma in eruptive cases (most commonly GI cancer).
  - A severe form of PCOS is HAIR-AN syndrome (**H**yper**A**ndrogenism, **I**nsulin **R**esistance, **A**canthosis **N**igricans).

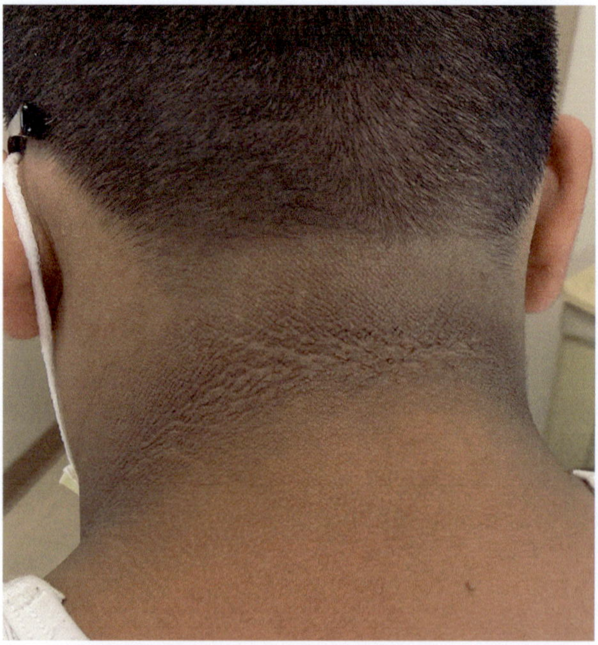

2. Acne vulgaris

- Morphology/clinical features
  - Open comedones (blackheads), closed comedones (whiteheads), inflammatory papules, inflammatory pustules, nodules, and cysts.
  - Lesions can coalesce into plaques and sinus tracts.
  - May see post-inflammatory hyperpigmentation and scars (icepick, rolling, boxcar, hypertrophic, and keloidal) as lesions resolve.
  - Acne variants
    - Acne conglobata—severe eruptive nodulocystic acne without systemic manifestations.
    - Acne mechanica—due to repeated friction and pressure.
    - Acne excoriée (de jeunes filles)—young women who pick at their acne, which leads to erosions, ulcerations, and scarring.
    - Neonatal acne—appears in first few weeks of life and usually resolves around 3 months, etiology is *Malassezia,* and treatment is ketoconazole cream.
    - Infantile acne—appears at 3–6 months and usually resolves around 2–3 years, similar to adolescent acne but must treat with traditional acne medications due to risk of scarring.
    - Acne cosmetica/pomade acne—due to cosmetics or greasy hair pomades.
    - Chloracne—occupational acne due to chlorinated aromatic hydrocarbons, very difficult to treat, and may have recurrent outbreaks.
    - Radiation acne—acne secondary to radiation therapy or other exposures (occupational, accidental).
- Distribution
  - Favors sebaceous areas including face, neck, upper chest, upper back and arms.
- Etiology/pathogenesis
  - Disease of the pilosebaceous that starts with abnormal follicular keratinization and has four main pathogenic processes.
    - Proliferation of *Cutibacterium acnes* (formerly known as *Propionibacterium acnes*), sebum overproduction from hormonal influences, abnormal keratinization, and inflammation.
    - Microcomedo is thought to be precursor lesion, rupture of a comedone leads to inflammation.
    - *Cutibacterium acnes* is a **gram-positive, anaerobic rod.**
- Internal sequelae/comorbidities
  - Usually none, may be associated with anxiety and depression.
  - Acne fulminans is a systemic disorder seen most commonly in males, 13–16 years old, which may be triggered by initiating isotretinoin or an increase in the dose.

    - Acute suppurative nodules, plaques with friable lesions and hemorrhagic crusts that can ulcerate and form black eschar.
    - Fever, increased WBC/ESR, and sterile osteolytic bone lesions.
    - Arthralgias, myalgias, and hepatosplenomegaly can be seen.
    - Treat with systemic steroids and slowly reintroduce and uptitrate isotretinoin.

  - Even mild acne can cause scarring.

- Laboratory testing

  - None.
  - If a "mid-childhood" acne case is seen (ages 1–7 years old), consider endocrine workup and bone age X-ray.
  - If PCOS is suspected (evidence of hirsutism and irregular menses), then check total/free testosterone, DHEAS, LH, and FSH.

- Treatments/prognosis

  - Refer to the following article from the American Academy of Dermatology (AAD): *Guidelines of care for the management of acne vulgaris. J Am Acad Dermatol 2024 May;90(5):1006.e1-1006.e30. doi 10.1016/j.jaad.2023.12.017.*
  - Topicals include clindamycin, tretinoin (retinoids), benzoyl peroxide wash, dapsone, azelaic acid, clascoterone, and salicylic acid.

    - Topicals work slowly.

  - Systemics include tetracyclines (doxy, mino, sare), spironolactone, OCPs, and isotretinoin.
  - Role of diet is controversial but skim milk, whey protein, and high glycemic load may contribute to acne.
  - Every single acne patient should be on a retinoid (oral or topical).
  - Do not use topical dapsone, it will not work.

- USMLE Board Review Pearls

  - Know the causes of an acneiform eruption which are (**Mnemonic: "SHIELD yourself from acne with Vitamin T**:" **S**teroids, **H**alogens, **I**soniazid, **E**GFR inhibitors, **L**ithium, **D**ilantin (phenytoin), **V**itamin B2, B6, B12, **T**estosterone).

    - This presents as monomorphic, inflammatory papules/pustules without comedones on the face and upper half of the body.

  - Know the pathogenesis of acne (see above).
  - Males usually have more severe acne due to greater androgen production.
  - Picking at acne scars can exacerbate scarring, must intervene with medications or behavioral therapy, and treat acne aggressively.

- Acne can be seen in congenital adrenal hyperplasia, PCOS, and Cushing syndrome.
- If mild to moderate acne, then start with topical medications; and if moderate to severe acne, can add a systemic agent.
- Severe and treatment-resistant acne (to all of the above therapies) should be treated with isotretinoin (chemical name: 13-*cis*-retinoic acid).

  - This medication is a teratogen and female patients must be abstinent from sex or use two forms of birth control while on the medication and require monthly pregnancy tests. There are no reproductive precautions in males who take isotretinoin because the amount of drug in the semen is negligible but they cannot donate blood (females cannot donate blood while on isotretinoin as well). A washout period of 1 month is required before getting pregnant or donating blood.
  - A recent Delphi consensus panel in *JAMA Dermatology* recommends checking only ALT and triglycerides before initiation and at peak dose (usually 2 months later) for patients on this medication (*Xia et. al. doi: 10.1001/jamadermatol.2022.2044*).
  - "Population-based studies have not identified an increased risk of neuropsychiatric conditions or inflammatory bowel disease (IBD) in patients with acne undergoing isotretinoin treatment" as per the above AAD Acne Management Guidelines.

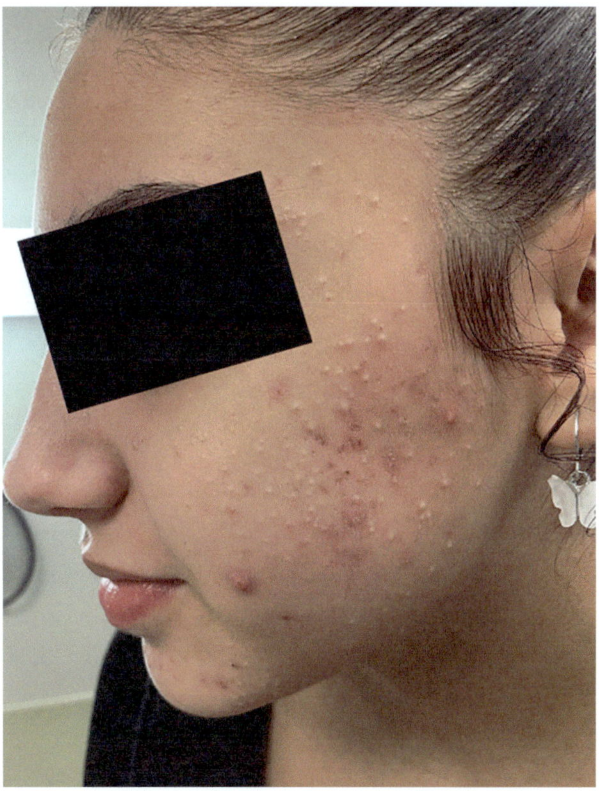

3. Actinic (solar) keratosis

- Morphology/clinical features
  - Scaly red papules.
  - These lesions are often better “felt” than “seen.”
    - They have a rough and hyperkeratotic feel.
  - Pigmented actinic keratoses are a subtype that lacks erythema and have a hyperpigmented or reticulated appearance.
  - Actinic cheilitis is a term used to describe actinic keratosis like changes on the lips, which presents as well-demarcated erythematous patches or thin plaques with scale on the mucosa/vermilion of the lips.
- Distribution
  - Sun-exposed areas.
    - Scalp, face, helices of the ear, dorsal hands, and forearms.
- Etiology/pathogenesis
  - UVB responsible through the induction of thymidine dimers.
  - p53 mutations within keratinocytes lead to impaired apoptosis.
- Internal sequelae/comorbidities
  - Patients with these lesions have a history of chronic sun exposure, so patients should be counseled to monitor for any changing or new suspicious skin lesions as well as the need for sun protection.
- Laboratory testing
  - None.
- Treatments/prognosis
  - Destructive measures
    - Cryosurgery.
  - Topical therapies
    - 5-FU (apply BID for 2–3 weeks for the face), imiquimod (use 5% TIW until they can’t tolerate it anymore), and tirbanibulin.
  - For diffuse or broad areas, consider field therapy with topical medications. Photodynamic therapy can also be used.
- USMLE Board Review Pearls
  - Rate of transformation to squamous cell carcinoma (SCC) is approximately 0.075–0.096% per year (some sources state a higher rate).
  - Lesions should be treated to prevent progression to SCC.

- Looks for characteristic lesions (erythematous lesions with "sandpaper" like scale that can become crusted) on sun-exposed areas in older patients, usually there will be a background of solar lentigines or solar purpura.
- If lesions are larger (usually > 1cm), then a biopsy is indicated to rule out SCC.
- Counsel patients on the need for sun protection.

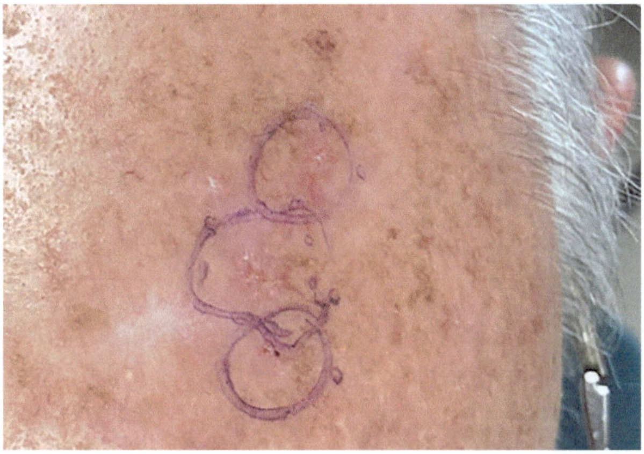

4. Alopecia areata

- Morphology/clinical features
  - Round or oval patches of nonscarring hair loss (the follicular ostia are visible).
  - Hair may regrow white.
  - Asymptomatic.
  - Can have **regular** nail pitting.
  - Alopecia areata (AA) variants.
    - Totalis—complete scalp hair loss.
    - Universalis—complete scalp and body hair loss.
    - Ophiasis pattern—band-like loss across occipital and temporal scalp.
    - Diffuse—widespread and **rapid** hair thinning/loss in one or more large areas, hair will come back: good prognosis!
- Distribution
  - Scalp.
  - Can also affect eyebrows, eyelashes, beard area, and genital hair.

- Etiology/pathogenesis
  - Loss of immune privilege with invasion of CD8+ T-cells targeting antigens in the hair follicle.
  - Genetics play a role.
- Internal sequelae/comorbidities
  - Associated with atopic dermatitis, autoimmune thyroid disease, vitiligo, lupus, and IBD.
- Laboratory testing
  - TSH.
- Treatments/prognosis
  - Topical therapies (very limited efficacy).
    - Corticosteroids, minoxidil, and topical allergens (squaric acid, DNCP, DPCP).
  - Intralesional corticosteroid injections work well but patients require repeat injections.
  - JAK inhibitors.
    - Baricitinib (JAK 1/2 inhibitor), ritlecitinib (JAK 3 and TEC kinase inhibitor) and deuruxolitinib (JAK1/2 inhibitor).
  - Good prognosis for a few spots and worse prognosis for extensive hair loss or persistent hair loss.
- USMLE Board Review Pearls
  - Look for completely round patches of hair loss on the scalp.
  - Nonscarring hair disease.
  - Patients are asymptomatic.
  - 25% of patients have a family history.
  - This is a CD8+ T-cell-mediated condition.
  - Baricitinib, ritlecitinib and deuruxolitinib are JAK inhibitors FDA approved to treat AA.
    - Baricitinib is also FDA approved to treat COVID-19 infections in hospitalized patients.

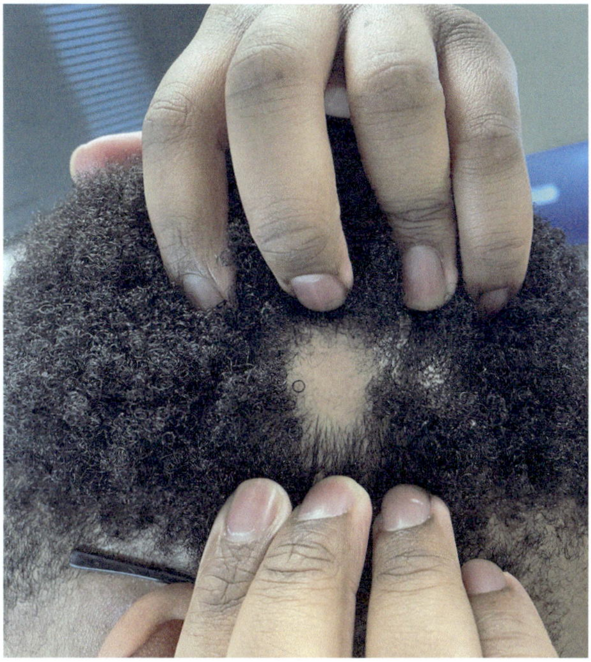

5. Androgenetic alopecia

- Morphology/clinical features
  - Males—frontotemporal recession and thinning over frontal crown and vertex scalp (Norwood–Hamilton classification).
  - Females—preservation of frontal hairline with progressive thinning from vertex to frontal scalp, thin and widened central part (Ludwig Scale).
- Distribution
  - Scalp.
- Etiology/pathogenesis
  - Genetic predisposition (polygenic).
  - In men—increased amount of dihydrotestosterone (DHT).
    - DHT is synthesized from testosterone by 5α-reductase.
- Internal sequelae/comorbidities
  - None.
- Laboratory testing
  - None.

- Treatments/prognosis
  - Topical
    - Minoxidil 2% or 5%.
  - Oral
    - Minoxidil, finasteride (males), and spironolactone (females).
  - Hair transplantation in chronic, stable cases.
  - Need to counsel patients on expectations of treatment.
    - A patient in their 20s or 30s with AGA will expect to get more hair regrowth with therapy than a patient in their 60s.
- USMLE Board Review Pearls
  - In the early phases of disease, this is a nonscarring hair loss.
  - 5α-reductase is the enzyme responsible for synthesizing DHT.
  - Finasteride is a type II 5α-reductase inhibitor and cannot be used in pregnant females due to the risk of abnormal male genitalia in the fetus.
  - Minoxidil was originally developed as a blood pressure medication but is now used in this condition because a side effect of the medication is hypertrichosis.

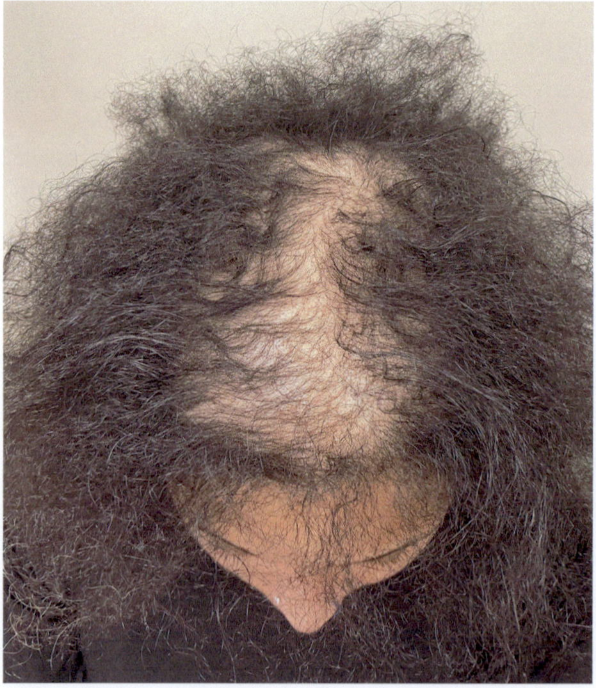

6. Atopic dermatitis (AD)

- Morphology/clinical features
  - Characterized by edematous, erythematous, papules and plaques which may exhibit vesiculation, oozing, scale, and serous crust.
  - Will likely see excoriations on normal and diseased skin.
  - Chronic lesions (seen more in adult forms) present as thickened plaques with lichenification and scale.
  - Pruritus is an essential feature.
- Distribution
  - Infantile AD—favors scalp, face, and extensor surfaces.
    - Diaper area is often spared.
  - Childhood AD—favors flexures and neck.
  - Adolescent/adult AD—favors flexures, face, neck, retroauricular, upper arms, back, and acral sites.
    - Often there is hand, wrist, and neck involvement.
- Etiology/pathogenesis
  - Complex interaction between epidermal barrier dysfunction, immune dysregulation, and environment.
    - Filaggrin mutations cause alteration in the epidermal barrier.
      - Leads to transepidermal water loss, xerosis, and entry of pathogens and microbes.
    - Upregulation of Th2 cytokines, including IL-4, IL-5, IL-12, and IL-13.
    - More than 90% of patients with AD have skin colonized by *staph aureus* (compared to 5% of unaffected patients).
      - Due to microbial dysbiosis in the affected skin.
- Internal sequelae/comorbidities
  - Patients usually have other "atopic" conditions such as allergic rhinitis or asthma.
  - Ocular comorbidities include allergic rhinoconjunctivitis, vernal keratoconjunctivitis, atopic keratoconjunctivitis, and keratoconus.
  - Increased risk of depression, anxiety, suicidal ideation, and sleep disturbances.
  - Emerging data points to cardiovascular complications including angina, MI, stroke, and heart failure but more research is needed.

- Laboratory testing
  - None.
- Treatments/prognosis
  - Topical therapies
    - Corticosteroids, calcineurin inhibitors, crisabarole (PDE-4 inhibitor), ruxolitinib (JAK 1/2 inhibitor), roflumilast (PDE-4 inhibitor), and tapinarof (aryl hydrocarbon receptor agonist).
  - Oral systemic therapies
    - Abrocitinib (JAK 1 inhibitor), upadacitinib (JAK 1 inhibitor), and corticosteroid taper.
  - Biologics
    - Dupilumab (blocks IL-4 and IL-13), tralokinumab (blocks IL-13), lebrikizumab (blocks IL-13), and nemolizumab (IL-31 receptor blocker).
- USMLE Board Review Pearls
  - Look for personal/family history of asthma, allergic rhinitis, and food allergies.
  - Triggers include climate, food, skin irritants, and allergens.
  - Know the manifestations of AD by age group.
    - Flexural involvement is a characteristic area.
  - Diagnosis is made by physical exam and HPI.
  - A primary goal of therapy is to break the itch/scratch cycle with medications to treat the symptoms of AD and xerosis (dry skin).
  - Topical corticosteroids are first-line therapy but are not for extended use given side effects and rebound flares, and medications like dupilumab are best for long-term disease control.
  - Must counsel patients to avoid harsh soaps, long and hot showers/baths and irritating clothing/fragrances, and to moisturize daily.
  - If a patient is not improving on biologic therapy for atopic dermatitis after many months, consider a skin biopsy to rule out mycosis fungoides (Cutaneous T-cell lymphoma).

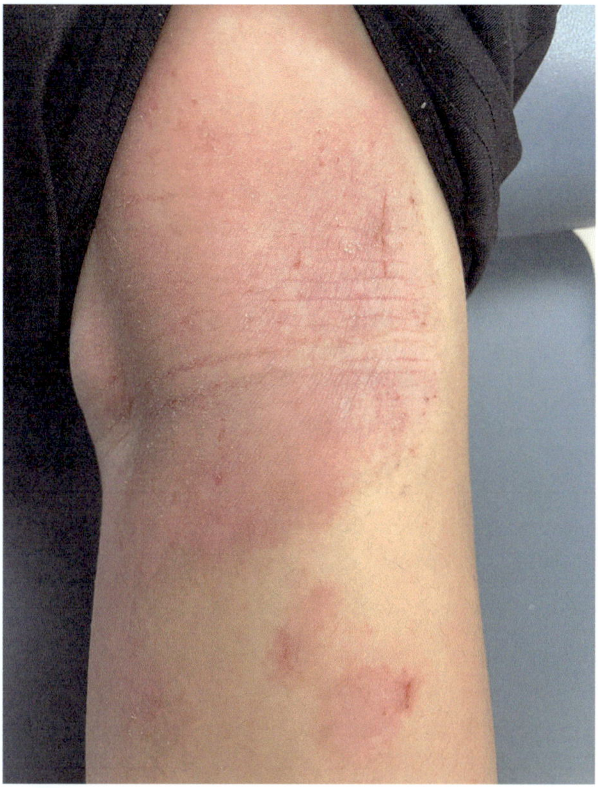

7. Basal cell carcinoma

- Morphology/clinical features
  - Well-circumscribed, pink/erythematous, macule/patch, or thin papule/plaque with focal scale or crust.
    - In more developed lesions, there may be a thin rolled border or ulceration.
    - Nodular basal cell carcinoma is described as a pink/red "pearly" papule with telangiectasias.
  - Morpheaform basal cell carcinoma is described as "scar-like" in appearance.
- Distribution
  - Most commonly seen on sun-exposed/sun-damaged skin.
    - Face, scalp, upper trunk, and upper extremities.

- Etiology/pathogenesis
  - UV radiation.
    - Intermittent, intense episodes of UV exposure and sunburns appear to increase the risk.
  - Genetic syndromes such as basal cell nevus syndrome, Bazex–Dupré–Christol, Rombo syndromes, and xeroderma pigmentosum.
- Internal sequelae/comorbidities
  - While metastasis of BCC is very rare, with an incidence rate of 0.0028–0.55%, it is still a possibility but usually it is in the case of very large, ulcerative, and neglected tumors.
- Laboratory testing
  - Skin biopsy.
    - There should be a low threshold to biopsy any pink papule in an older sun-damaged patient.
- Treatments/prognosis
  - Surgical treatments are standard of care and include wide local excision, Mohs surgery, and ED&C.
  - Systemic treatments
    - Vismodegib and sonidegib (hedgehog pathway inhibitors), cemiplimab (PD-1 inhibitor).
  - Topical therapy (superficial BCC)
    - 5-FU and imiquimod.
- USMLE Board Review Pearls
  - Most common malignant skin cancer; nodular form accounts for nearly 80% of BCCs.
  - A locally destructive tumor with a very low metastatic potential.
  - Main risk factor is sun exposure.
  - Multiple BCCs that appear early in life on non-sun-exposed areas are suggestive of a genetic syndrome (such as basal cell nevus syndrome a.k.a. Gorlin syndrome).
  - Mohs surgery is the treatment of choice for cosmetically sensitive areas or where tissue-sparing surgery is important (such as the pre-tibial area).

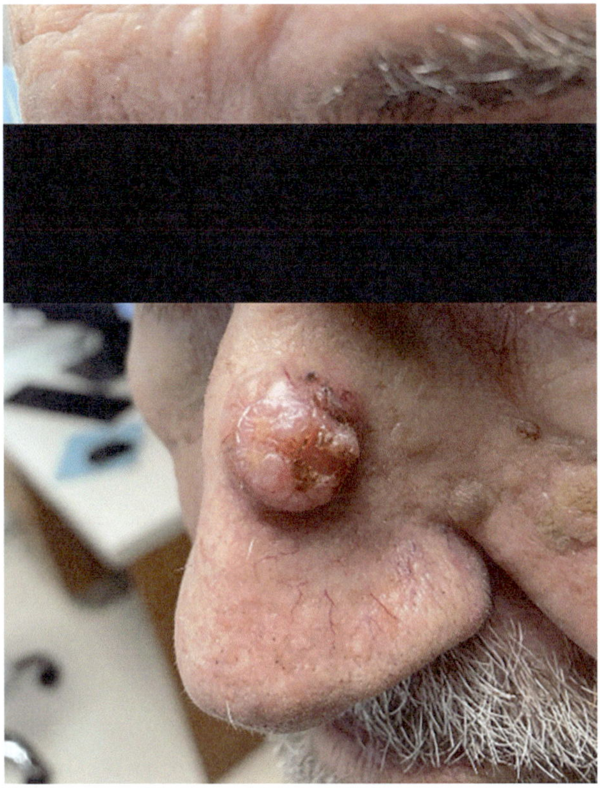

8. Bedbugs
   - Morphology/clinical features
     - Erythematous/urticarial grouped papules at bite sites.
       - Usually, bites are in groups of 2–3, which is called the "breakfast, lunch, and dinner sign."
       - Sometimes there is a central hemorrhagic punctum.
     - Mild pruritus associated with bites.
   - Distribution
     - Commonly on the trunk and extremities and other exposed areas.

- Etiology/pathogenesis
  - The scientific name for bedbugs is *Cimex lectularius.*
  - *Cimex hemipterus* is a type of bedbug that primarily resides in tropical climates.
  - Bedbug bite reactions result from an immune response to salivary proteins (e.g., nitrophorin) injected by the insect while feeding.
- Internal sequelae/comorbidities
  - None.
  - To date, transmission of infectious diseases to humans by bedbugs has not been documented.
- Laboratory testing
  - None.
- Treatments/prognosis
  - Can treat the pruritus with topical steroids or topical antihistamines.
  - Ultimately the infestation needs to be eradicated by a professional exterminator or the patient will continue to be impacted.
- USMLE Board Review Pearls
  - Look for erythematous papules in groups of three (this is characteristic of many arthropod assaults).
  - Transmitted by contact with infested bedding but also by infested furniture such as couches or chairs. Hotels are commonly affected and there are even cases of movie theatre seats becoming infested.
  - The bites will resolve in 1–2 weeks but the infestation must be eradicated at its source; treating the skin of the patient in the office is not good enough.
  - Bedbugs can be seen with the naked eye and are the size of apple seeds.
  - Bedbugs often hide in the seams, folds, and tags of mattresses and may not be readily apparent upon a cursory glance.

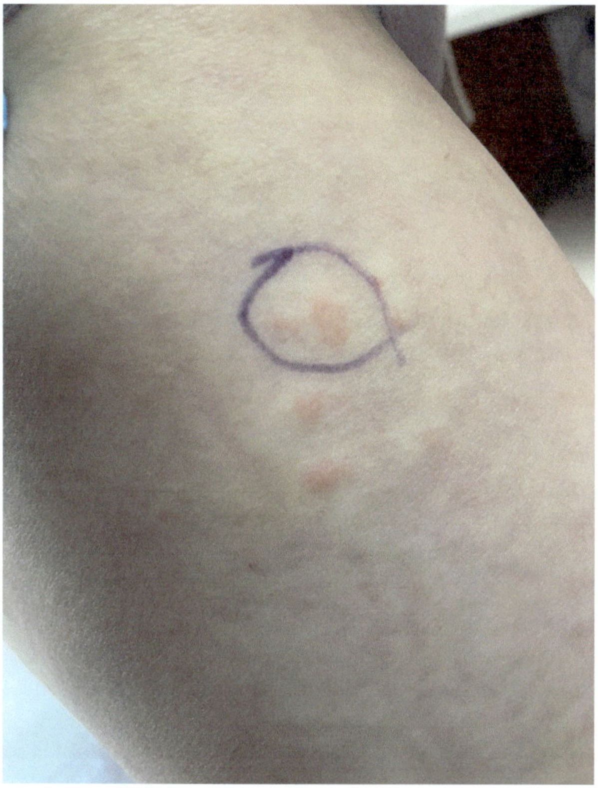

9. Bullous pemphigoid

- Morphology/clinical features
  - Nonbullous (early phase)—persistent, polymorphous eruption that presents with isolated and intensely pruritic fixed urticarial papules and plaques (sometimes annular in configuration).
  - Bullous phase—tense, fluid-filled vesicles and bullae (clear/tan > blood tinged) on the background of an urticarial plaque.
- Distribution
  - Commonly affects trunk, abdomen, flexural, and fold areas.
- Etiology/pathogenesis
  - IgG autoantibodies bind hemidesmosome proteins, which causes complement activation leading to degradation and destruction of anchoring proteins leading to a subepidermal blister (type II hypersensitivity reaction).

  - The most important target antigen is the noncollagenous NC16A domain of BP180 (a.k.a. BPAG2, type XVII collagen).
    - The secondary target is BP230 (BPAG1), which is affected through epitope spreading.
- Internal sequelae/comorbidities
  - None.
- Laboratory testing
  - BPAGs (test serum of patient with ELISA technique to detect circulating antibodies to BP180 and BP230).
- Treatments/prognosis
  - Mild disease
    - Tetracycline + nicotinamide.
    - Superpotent topical steroid.
  - Moderate to severe disease
    - Systemic steroids with a slower taper over 6–9 months.
    - Steroid-sparing immunosuppressives (MMF, MTX, azathioprine). Dupilumab is FDA approved for use with a tapering course of PO corticosteroids.
    - IVIg (don't forget to check IgA levels before administering).
- USMLE Board Review Pearls
  - Most common autoimmune blistering disease (affecting patients 60 years of age and older), where the blister is located in the basement membrane zone.
  - Patients will report severe pruritus.
  - The bullae can be small but are always tense.
  - Autoantibodies are against hemidesmosomes specifically BPAG1 and BPAG2.
  - Look for firm yellow-tinged blisters on an urticarial base.
  - Mucosal involvement and mortality are possible but rare. This is not a dangerous disease in terms of mortality.
  - The direct immunofluorescence of BP will show linear pattern at dermal–epidermal junction and the H&E will show many eosinophils.
  - Nikolsky sign is negative.
  - The best test for BP is a direct immunofluorescence; if this test is negative, then the diagnosis is not BP.
  - If a patient has BP for more than 6 months and is not improving on treatment, then consider a salt split skin test to ensure that the patient does not have a different blistering disease.
    - BP should be relatively easy to treat.

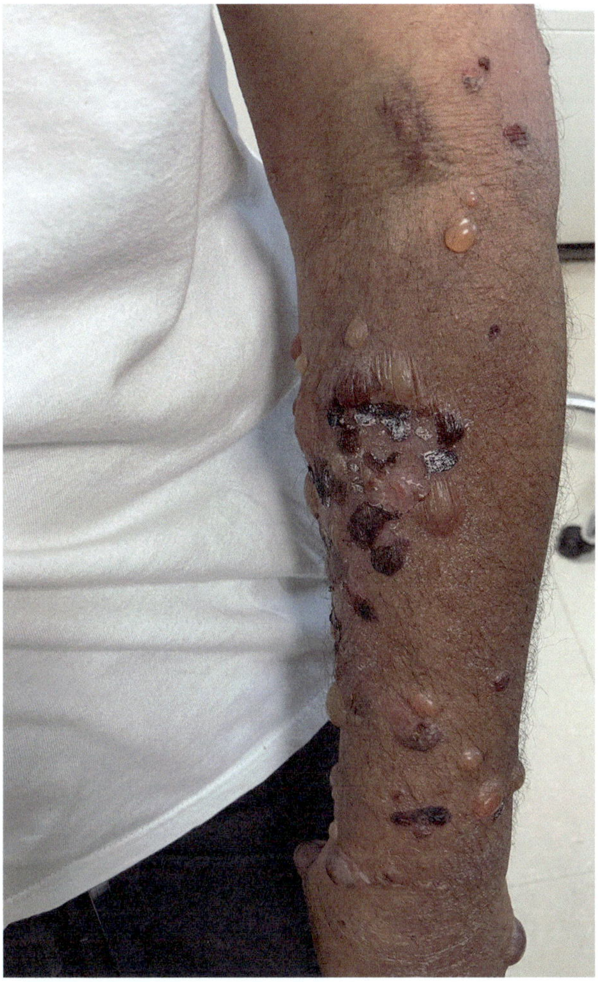

10. Calciphylaxis

- Morphology/clinical features
  - Painful and stellate or retiform purpuric plaques that can progress to indurated, necrotic, and ulcerative plaques.
- Distribution
  - Commonly seen on lower legs and abdomen.
- Etiology/pathogenesis
  - Due to small-medium vessel calcification and thrombosis from calcium deposit in the vessels.
  - Most commonly occurs in the setting of ESRD due to an increase in calcium phosphate production.

  - In some cases, can also occur due to diabetes mellitus and hyperparathyroidism.
- Internal sequelae/comorbidities
  - Secondary infections and sepsis.
  - High mortality rate.
- Laboratory testing
  - Bone scintigraphy has been reported to have a 97% specificity rate and 89% sensitivity rate for diagnosing calciphylaxis.
- Treatments/prognosis
  - Treat underlying renal failure with low calcium dialysis.
  - Sodium thiosulfate with dialysis.
  - Treat and manage underlying infections.
- USMLE Board Review Pearls
  - Look for stellate necrotic plaques on the legs or abdomen in a renal failure patient on dialysis (or other areas of high adipose tissue density).
  - Early recognition and treatment are imperative because secondary infection and sepsis can develop as well as internal organ involvement.

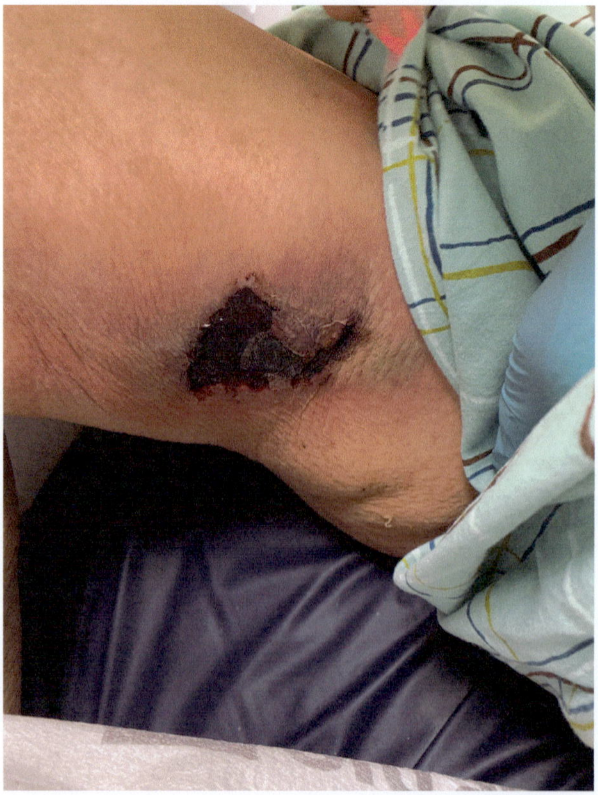

11. Candidiasis

- Morphology/clinical features/distribution
  - Mucous membrane candidiasis
    - White "cottage-cheese"-like plaques in the vaginal mucosa or oral cavity. Patients with vaginal candidiasis may report burning, dysuria, and pruritus. Oral candidiasis is painless and is easily scrapped off with a tongue depressor revealing erythema and erosions (helpful clue on physical exam).
    - Median rhomboid glossitis is a candidal infection of the oral cavity manifested by a central smooth erythema of the tongue.
    - Angular cheilitis (perlèche) is a candidal infection of the corners of the mouth manifested by moist, macerated erythematous plaques with erosions, angular fissures, and soreness.
  - Cutaneous candidiasis
    - Candidal intertrigo is a candida infection of the skin folds manifested by beefy red plaques with satellite pustules.
      - Commonly seen in the inframammary folds and in the groin.
    - Erosio interdigitalis blastomycetica is a candidal infection manifested by a moist, macerated, erythematous plaque classically in the third web space of the fingers.
  - Deep fungal infection
    - Seen in immunosuppressed patients who are neutropenic manifested by scattered papules/nodules that progress to hemorrhagic and necrotic plaques.
- Etiology/pathogenesis
  - Species is *Candida albicans* (most common in localized and systemic infections).
    - Another cause is *C. tropicalis.*
  - Secretory aspartyl proteinases (SAPs) and phospholipases aid in fungal adhesion and tissue invasion.
- Internal sequelae/comorbidities
  - Risk factors include DM2, corticosteroids, and immunosuppression.
  - Deep fungal infections have a 30% mortality rate and usually begin in GI tract and may also infect the muscles, retina, heart valve, and other internal organs.

- Laboratory testing
  - KOH prep will show yeast and pseudohyphae.
  - Fungal culture/blood culture.
- Treatments/prognosis
  - Topical treatments include nystatin and clotrimazole.
  - Oral treatments include fluconazole.
  - Amphotericin B, azoles, and echinocandins for systemic infections.
  - Keep skin folds clean and dry; this disease is worsened by sweating and occlusion.
- USMLE Board Review Pearls
  - The most common species to cause infection is *C. albicans* and usually leads to thrush or yeast infection clinically.
  - A dimorphic species that forms pseudohyphae and budding yeasts at 20°C and germ tubes at 37°C.
  - Look for eroded and erythematous papules and plaques in skin folds such as groin, axilla, vagina, and below the breasts.
  - Patients usually have a history of antibiotic use, steroid use, diabetes, or immunosuppression.
  - Candidal esophagitis is seen in patients with hematologic malignancies or AIDS.
  - Diagnosis can be made from skin exam findings and history.
  - The most accurate test is a blood culture.
  - Chronic mucocutaneous candidiasis is a genetic disorder due to a mutation in *AIRE,* which leads to T-cell dysfunction and impaired immunity against *C. albicans.*
  - Know how to treat the different forms of a candidal infection.
    - Oral candidiasis—PO fluconazole tablets, nystatin swish and swallow, and clotrimazole troches.
    - Esophageal candidiasis—systemic fluconazole, echinocandins, and amphotericin B.
    - Superficial (cutaneous) candidiasis—topical antifungals, keep skin clean and dry with powder-based vehicles.
    - Vulvovaginal candidiasis—topical antifungal, single dose of oral fluconazole.
    - Diaper rash—topical nystatin.

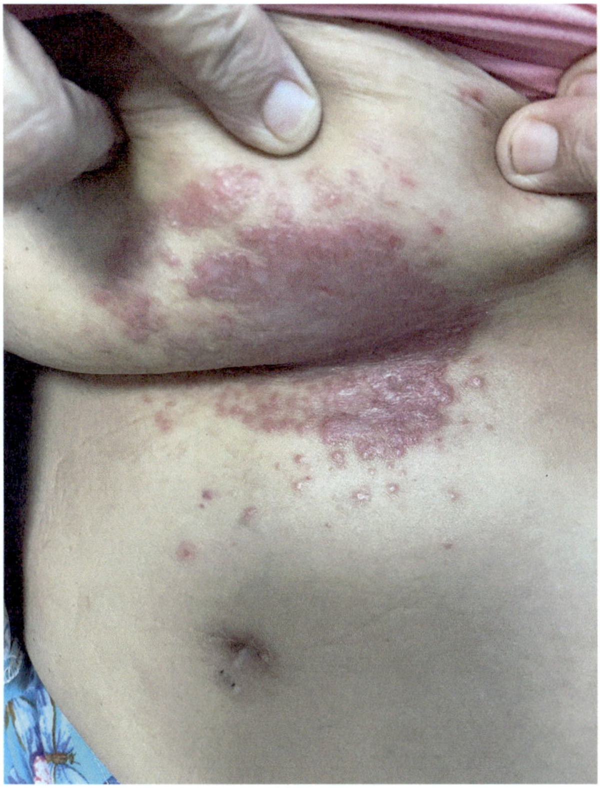

12. Carcinoma en cuirasse (carcinoma erysipeloides)

    - Morphology/clinical features
        - Carcinoma en cuirasse—indurated, leathery skin with orange peel-like (peau d'orange) appearance and feel.
        - Carcinoma erysipeloides—well-demarcated, raised erythematous plaque.
        - Demonstrates "sclerodermoid" skin changes.
    - Distribution
        - Chest wall/breast.
    - Etiology/pathogenesis
        - Due to metastatic carcinoma infiltrating the lymphatic vessels.
    - Internal sequelae/comorbidities
        - Secondary to metastatic breast cancer.
        - Breast cancer is the most common cause but can be seen with other cancers.

- Laboratory testing
  - Skin biopsy.
- Treatments/prognosis
  - Treat underlying breast cancer.
  - Poor prognosis.
- USMLE Board Review Pearls
  - Look for a large leathery, indurated, and peau d'orange plaque overlying the chest wall/breast.
  - There will likely be a mastectomy scar, indicating the patient has a history of breast cancer.
  - Patient needs prompt referral to a breast oncologist.

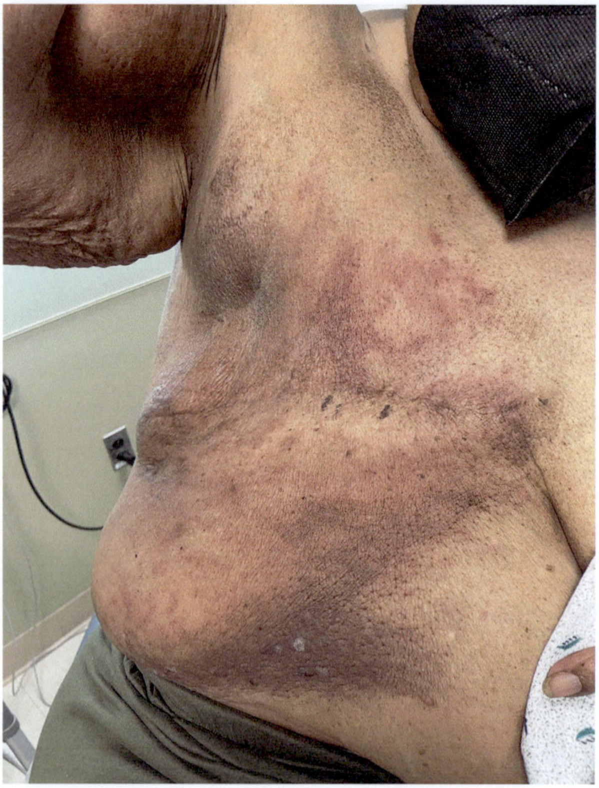

13. Central centrifugal cicatricial alopecia (CCCA)

- Morphology/clinical features
  - Smooth, scarred areas without visibility of the follicular ostia.
  - Destructive, chronic, and progressive hair loss.
  - Baby doll hairs are present (polytrichia, in which multiple hairs emerge from a single follicular opening).
  - Patients may complain of mild pruritus, pain, and tenderness.
  - The earliest signs of disease are peri-pilar halo and polytrichia.
- Distribution
  - Scarring starts on vertex, then spreads centrifugally over time.
- Etiology/pathogenesis
  - Traditionally associated with chemical relaxers, hot combs, traumatic hairstyles, and pomades in female patients of African descent.
  - Genetic predisposition with mutation in *PADI3* in some patients.
- Internal sequelae/comorbidities
  - None.
- Laboratory testing
  - None.
- Treatments/prognosis
  - Tetracyclines for pain, pruritus, and tenderness.
  - Topical or intralesional corticosteroids.
  - Minoxidil for hair regrowth.
- USMLE Board Review Pearls
  - Look for a female patient of African descent who complains of mild tenderness and pain on the vertex of the scalp.
  - Must counsel patients to stop traumatic hair care practices, that there is no cure for this condition and the goal of therapy is to mitigate symptoms. Some patients may notice mild hair regrowth with therapy but eventually the scarring will progress.

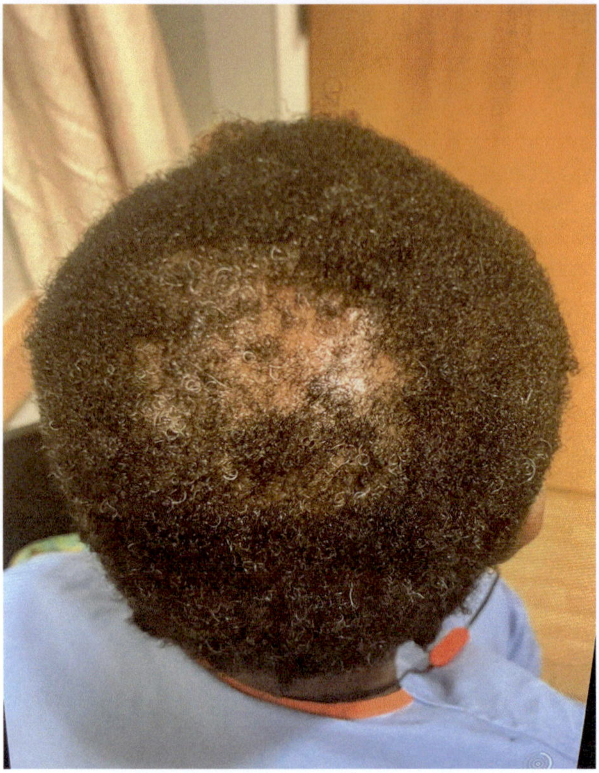

14. Cellulitis

- Morphology/clinical features
  - Tender/erythematous/warm ill-defined plaques.
  - Some patients present with fever/chills and lymphangitis.
  - Severe cases may present with necrosis, bullae, and vesicles.
- Distribution
  - Extremities in adults.
  - Head and neck in children.

- Etiology/pathogenesis
  - Skin infection due to *S. aureus* or group A *strep* of the deep dermis and sub-cutis.
- Internal sequelae/comorbidities
  - Often preceded by fever, chills, and malaise.
- Laboratory testing
  - None.
  - Blood cultures are almost always negative in immunocompetent patients.
- Treatments/prognosis
  - Uncomplicated cases
    - Oral dicloxacillin, cephalexin, or clindamycin.
  - A/w diabetic/decubitus ulcers
    - Piperacillin/tazobactam or ciprofloxacin + metronidazole.
  - Severe cases require hospitalization and IV antibiotics.
  - MRSA cellulitis must be treated with TMP/SMX, doxycycline, or clindamycin (presence of an abscess or necrotizing cellulitis is a clue).
- USMLE Board Review Pearls
  - Infection of the dermis and sub-cutis commonly due to *staph* or group A *strep* bacteria from a break in the skin or a systemic source.
  - Risk factors for cellulitis include diabetes, IV drug abuse, venous stasis, and immunosuppression.
  - Associated abscess, necrotizing cellulitis, or purulent cellulitis is likely due to MRSA cellulitis and must be treated with TMP/SMX, doxycycline, or clindamycin.
  - Clinical exam is sufficient for diagnosis.
  - Topical antibiotics are ineffective because this is a deeper infection.
  - PO antibiotics should be given for 5–10 days. IV antibiotics are indicated if there is evidence of systemic toxicity, diabetes, and extremes of age or hand/orbital involvement.

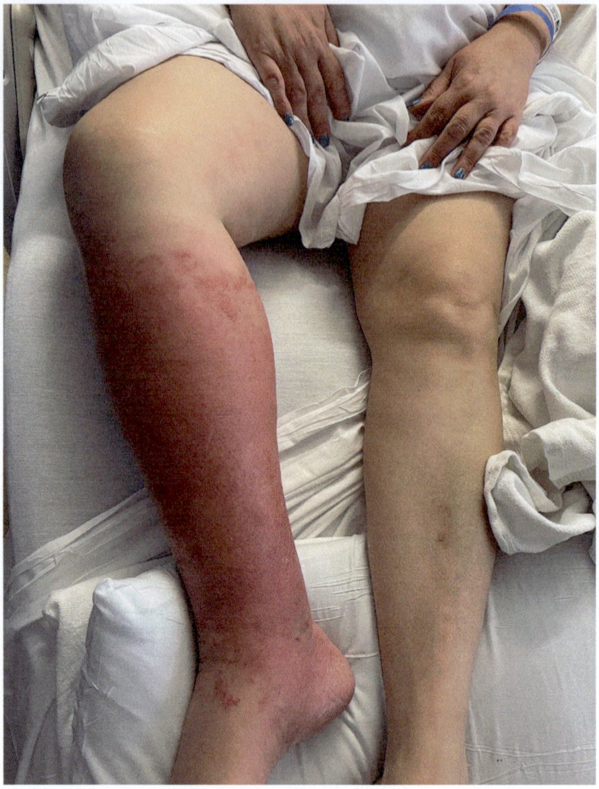

15. Cherry angioma (cherry hemangioma)

- Morphology/clinical features
  - Round to oval, bright red to purple, dome-shaped papule ranging in size from pinpoint to several millimeters.
    - May appear multilobulated in larger lesions.
- Distribution
  - Common on the trunk and extremities.
- Etiology/pathogenesis
  - Acquired cutaneous vascular proliferation.
  - Somatic mutations in three *GNA* genes—*GNA11, GNA14,* and *GNAQ*—have been identified in the majority of cherry angiomas.
  - Hormonal factors may play a role.

- Internal sequelae/comorbidities
  - None.
- Laboratory testing
  - None.
- Treatments/prognosis
  - Shave excision, electrodessication, and laser ablation.
- USMLE Board Review Pearls
  - Look for small, vascular, red papules appearing anywhere on the body.
  - Most common benign vascular tumor and frequency increases with age.
  - No treatment is necessary but can be removed for cosmetic reasons.
  - These do not regress spontaneously (as opposed to infantile hemangiomas).
  - Also known as benign capillary hemangioma.

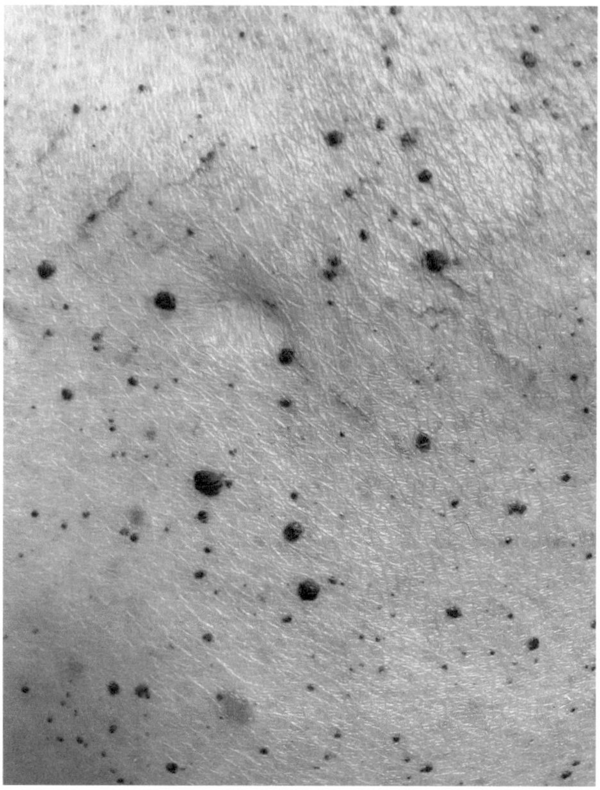

16. Chondrodermatitis nodularis helicis

- Morphology/clinical features
  - Tender, pink, crusted papule.
  - **Painful**.
- Distribution
  - Cartilaginous portion of helix and anti-helix of the ear.
    - Upper helix the number 1 site in males and anti-helix number 1 site in females.
- Etiology/pathogenesis
  - Not completely known but likely due to a combination of chronic pressure, ischemia, actinic damage, and cold exposure leading to inflammation.
- Internal sequelae/comorbidities
  - None.
- Laboratory testing
  - None.
- Treatments/prognosis
  - Specially designed pillows or padding to relieve pressure.
  - Surgical methods such as shave excision or cryosurgery.
  - Intralesional steroids.
- USMLE Board Review Pearls
  - Initial therapy should be counseling and offloading of pressure with specially designed pillows or padding (as a general rule of thumb for exam questions, start with the most noninvasive or benign therapy first if appropriate in the given context).
  - If there is a high level of suspicion (i.e., lesion has been rapidly growing), the lesion should be biopsied to rule out a skin cancer.

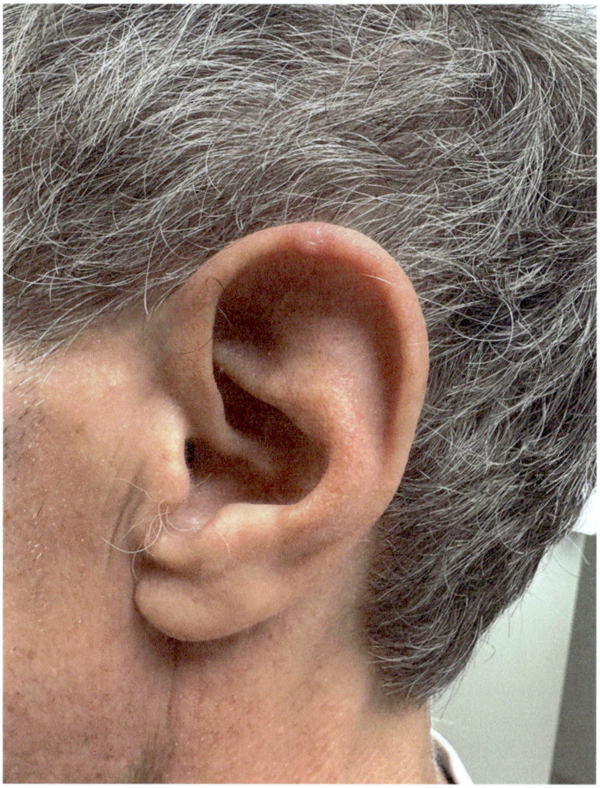

17. Congenital melanocytic nevus

    - Morphology/clinical features

        - Nevus that is present at birth that begins as a tan papule or plaque and progressively darkens over the first year of life.
        - May also develop hypertrichosis and "proliferative nodules."
        - Some may have a pebbly surface and appearance.
        - Characterized by size

            - Small is < 1.5 cm.
            - Medium is 1.5–19.9 cm.
            - Large is > 20 cm.
            - Giant > 40 cm.

- Distribution
  - Anywhere but commonly seen on the trunk and extremities.
- Etiology/pathogenesis
  - *NRAS* mutation in a majority of cases.
- Internal sequelae/comorbidities
  - Neurocutaneous melanosis/melanocytosis
    - Large/giant congenital melanocytic nevus are a/w benign or malignant melanocytic proliferation in leptomeninges and brain parenchyma.
    - Variable clinical presentation but in symptomatic patients there is a high morbidity and mortality from mass effect.
    - Screening with MRI is recommended with large posterior axial congenital nevus with multiple satellite nevi or multiple nevi (≥ 3 small to medium size but usually 10-20+).
  - The risk of melanoma in small/medium lesions is less than 1% and in giant nevi the risk is 5% (some sources state different rates).
    - Majority develop melanoma in the first 5 years of life.
    - Signs of rapid growth, induration, and ulceration should raise suspicion for melanoma within a congenital melanocytic nevus but mild change is normal.
    - Suspected proliferating nodules should be evaluated by biopsy.
- Laboratory testing
  - None.
- Treatments/prognosis
  - Surgical resection for cosmetic reasons for small to medium lesions.
  - Serial exams with photographs and measurements for large lesions.
  - If large/giant nevi are to be excised, patients should have a plastic surgery referral beginning after the patient is 6 months of age (delay excision in the case of symptomatic neurocutaneous melanosis).
- USMLE Board Review Pearls
  - Benign proliferation with an increased density of hair follicles.
  - Commonly presents as a solitary hyperpigmented lesion with coarse hair.
  - Know when to suspect and screen for neurocutaneous melanosis.
    - Look for large or giant congenital melanocytic nevus on the trunk with satellite lesions, especially if the patient has neurological signs or symptoms.

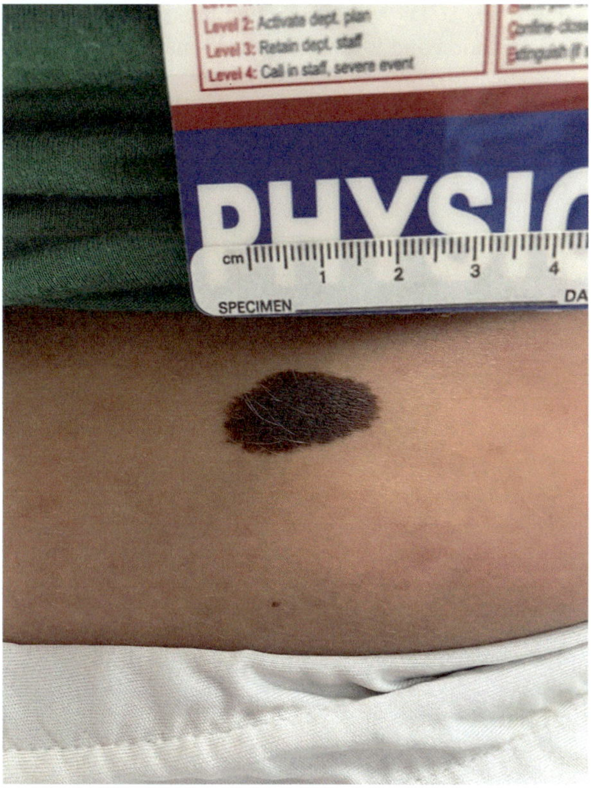

18. Contact dermatitis

- Morphology/clinical features
  - Irritant contact dermatitis (ICD)
    - Accounts for 80% of contact dermatitis cases. The most common cause of occupational skin disease.
      - Acute ICD—vesiculation/necrosis that has more clearly defined margins.
      - Chronic ICD—dryness, scaling, lichenification, and fissuring with ill-defined margins.
      - Can see pustular/acneiform ICD from metals, croton oil, mineral oils, tars, greases, cutting, and metal working fluids.
    - Allergic contact dermatitis (ACD)
      - Acute ACD—erythema/edema/papules/oozing/vesiculation in sharp demarcated pattern.

  - Chronic ACD—marked lichenification/fissuring/scaling with no vesiculation and less well-defined margins.

- Distribution
  - Distribution depends on the type of exposure.
    - ICD
      - Hands are the most common site, and face is the second most common site.
      - Airborne ICD involves the upper eyelids, philtrum, and submental region.
    - ACD
      - Linear streaks/vesicles on extremities—poison ivy (rhus dermatitis).
      - Fingertips in florists—flowers (tulips number 1).
      - Neck, cheeks, and postauricular—hair dyes (scalp is relatively resistant to ACD).
      - Periocular/eyelid—nail products (tosylamide) and cosmetics (false eyelashes, adhesives).
      - Lips—gallates, dyes, flavorings, and propolis (found in some lip balms).
      - Earlobe—nickel.
      - Neck—fragrances.
      - Wrist—chromates (leather).
      - Hands—gloves.
      - Spares axillary vault—clothing dermatitis.
      - Perianal—preservatives (MCI/MI).
      - Feet (spares toe webs)—shoe dermatitis from adhesives (colophony) and rubber accelerators (mercaptobenothiazole).
      - Ulcers—bacitracin, neomycin, and lanolin.
      - Airborne ACD—usually from plants (*Compositae* is number 1).
- Etiology/pathogenesis
  - ICD
    - Direct damage of keratinocytes by irritant, NOT immune-mediated and does NOT require previous sensitization.
      - A very common cause of chronic ICD on the hands is repetitive hand washing.
        - Removes lipid and water-retaining substances from mild irritants (soap/water), which leads to epidermal turnover/transepidermal water loss and inflammation.
      - Another very common cause is ICD from saliva = "lip licker's dermatitis."

  - ACD
    - Immune-mediated, delayed type IV hypersensitivity reaction.
    - Initial sensitization to allergen is required.
- Internal sequelae/comorbidities
  - Autosensitization (id reaction and disseminated eczema)
    - Secondary eczematous lesions develop in distant site from primary exposure appearing days to weeks later.
    - Possibly related to hematogenous dissemination of allergens or circulating activated memory T-cells.
    - Presents as ill-defined, symmetrical, eczematous areas in analogous anatomic sites.
- Laboratory testing
  - Patch testing for ACD
    - TRUE test (truetest.com)—three panels of 12 allergens.
    - Patch test results must be interpreted in the clinical context of the patient's presentation and must be relevant!
- Treatments/prognosis
  - Education and avoidance of allergen or irritant.
  - Topical corticosteroids/PO corticosteroid taper.
  - For ICD, many cases resolve spontaneously due to "hardening" phenomenon.
    - Skin adapts to the cause of ICD, resulting in a diminished response to the irritant.
  - After an acute ACD exposure like poison ivy, the involved area should be first washed with water—then soap can be considered. Consider PO steroid taper over 2–3 weeks (prednisone 60 mg, 40 mg, 20 mg for 5 days each).
- USMLE Board Review Pearls
  - Allergic contact dermatitis is a type IV hypersensitivity reaction that results from contact with a substance that the patient has been previously exposed to and it is more common in adults.
  - Look for nickel, poison ivy/oak, perfumes/deodorants, cosmetics, and neomycin (and other over-the-counter antibiotics) in the question stem or HPI and look for eczematous eruptions that often mirror the contact event.
  - Often described as a "linear," "angular," or "patterned" rash.
  - Best initial therapy is corticosteroids and allergen avoidance. Patch testing can be used after the acute eruption resolves to help narrow down the culprit or prove to the patient that a specific allergen is causing their dermatitis.

– Patch testing results are affected by topical steroids and topical calcineurin inhibitors (because they inhibit and treat inflammation). Antihistamines will not affect patch testing results because the type IV hypersensitivity reaction is not histamine related (i.e., patients do not need to stop antihistamines before and during patch testing).

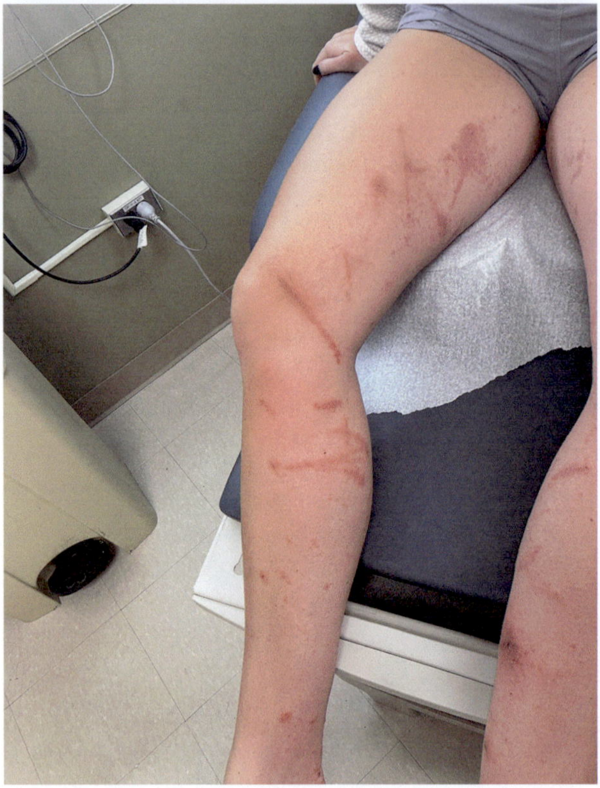

19. Cutaneous larva migrans

- Morphology/clinical features
  - Erythematous, serpiginous, cord-like, cutaneous eruption.
  - This creeping eruption moves 1–3 cm/day.
  - Patients may complain of pruritus.
- Distribution
  - Usually on feet.
- Etiology/pathogenesis
  - Organism found in animal feces.
  - The most common organism is *Ancylostoma braziliense.*

        - Also due to *A. caninum.*
- Internal sequelae/comorbidities
    - None.
        - The parasite penetrates the intact epidermis on the foot but is unable to penetrate the human basement membrane zone and therefore unable to cause systemic disease.
- Laboratory testing
    - None.
- Treatments/prognosis
    - Albendazole, ivermectin, and thiabendazole.
- USMLE Board Review Pearls
    - Look for the characteristic creeping eruption on the foot in a patient with a travel history. Patients will report walking barefoot on grass or sand.
    - Patients may complain of pruritus.
    - This is the most common tropical parasitic skin disease.

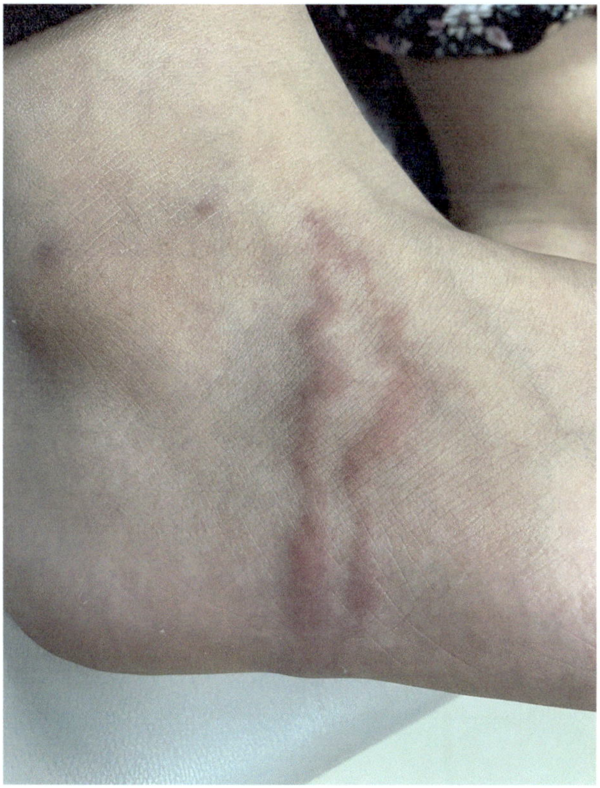

20. Cutaneous lupus erythematosus

- Morphology/clinical features/distribution
  - Acute cutaneous lupus erythematosus (ACLE)—malar erythema classically sparing the nasolabial folds (because these are "sun-protected" areas) commonly referred to as the "butterfly rash."
  - Subacute cutaneous lupus erythematosus (SCLE)—psoriasiform plaques or scaly polycyclic annular plaques with central clearing on sun-exposed areas such as neck, V-chest, and upper back/upper extremities.
    - Neonatal lupus erythematosus—subtype of SCLE in mothers who are anti-Ro/SS-A positive, neonates present with SCLE-like lesions favoring the face and periorbital area.
      - Risk of heart block, hepatobiliary disease, and hematologic abnormalities in the infant.
    - An erythema multiforme like presentation of SCLE is called "Rowell's syndrome." This is **NOT** a concurrent presentation of both erythema multiforme and cutaneous lupus.
  - Discoid lupus erythematosus—begins with erythematous macules or plaques that progress to lesions with scale, atrophy and scarring with central hypopigmentation and peripheral hyperpigmentation typically appearing on the scalp (associated with scarring alopecia) and ears (conchal bowl).
    - It is rare to have DLE lesions below the neck without head/neck involvement.
  - Chilblain lupus erythematosus—red or dusky purple plaques/papules on fingertips, helical rims, calves, and heels that are persistent.
  - Lupus panniculitis—indurated, nontender, subcutaneous nodules that heal with fat atrophy and appear indented on the upper outer arms, upper trunk, breasts, outer things, and buttocks.
    - Lupus panniculitis with overlying skin changes is referred to as Lupus profundus.
  - Tumid lupus erythematosus—edematous, nonscaly, erythematous often annular plaques on the face and trunk.
  - Bullous systemic lupus erythematosus—widespread, symmetric eruption of tense subepidermal bullae on an erythematous to urticarial base.
    - By definition, patients must meet the American College of Rheumatology (ACR) definition of systemic lupus erythematosus (SLE).
    - Antibodies are against type VII collagen.

- Etiology/pathogenesis
  - Varies but general principle is that SLE is an autoimmune disease where an environmental trigger (such as UV radiation) causes cellular and DNA damage with a concurrent defect in the phagocytic function of monocytes and macrophages that leads to loss of immune tolerance, which results in release of proinflammatory cytokines and production of autoantibodies that attack both normal and abnormal cells in the body.
- Internal sequelae/comorbidities
  - Every form of cutaneous lupus may be seen in the setting of SLE or as an isolated cutaneous disease. Below is a brief list of forms of cutaneous lupus and their association with SLE (i.e., the more * means a higher chance of a patient having SLE).
  - Acute cutaneous lupus (ACLE)—****.
  - Subacute cutaneous lupus erythematosus (SCLE)—***.
  - Discoid lupus erythematosus—*.
  - Chilblain lupus erythematosus—**.
  - Lupus panniculitis—*.
  - Tumid lupus erythematosus—controversial if this form is even associated with SLE at all.
  - Bullous systemic lupus erythematosus—***** (by definition patient has SLE).
- Laboratory testing
  - ANA, anti-Ro/SSA, and anti-LA/SSB.
- Treatments/prognosis
  - All lupus patients should be counseled on smoking cessation and sun protection.
  - Most forms of cutaneous lupus can be treated with antimalarials.
  - Treat underlying SLE if present.
  - The treatment of choice for bullous SLE is dapsone.
- USMLE Board Review Pearls
  - The classic question stem for a patient with SLE is as follows: a female of reproductive age presents with arthritis, cytopenia, fever, and a "butterfly rash."
  - Know which forms of cutaneous lupus are highly associated with SLE.
  - The medications that cause drug-induced SLE are hydralazine, procainamide, and quinidine.
  - SCLE can be drug induced, and the medications implicated are HCTZ, omeprazole, terbinafine, diltiazem, ACE inhibitors, nifedipine, and griseofulvin (mnemonic **HOT DANG**).
  - Bullous lupus = antibodies to collagen VII, treat with dapsone.
  - The rash of ACLE spares the nasolabial folds a.k.a. the "butterfly rash" (think of a butterfly flying away from the folds).

    - Nearly every patient on the exam or in the clinic who presents with a rash like this should have their ANA checked.

  - Patients who start on hydroxychloroquine for cutaneous lupus need a baseline eye examination and a follow-up exam to monitor for retinopathy that can be irreversible.
  - Tumid lupus is classically photoinduced but may not appear for 1–2 weeks and is usually seen in smokers.

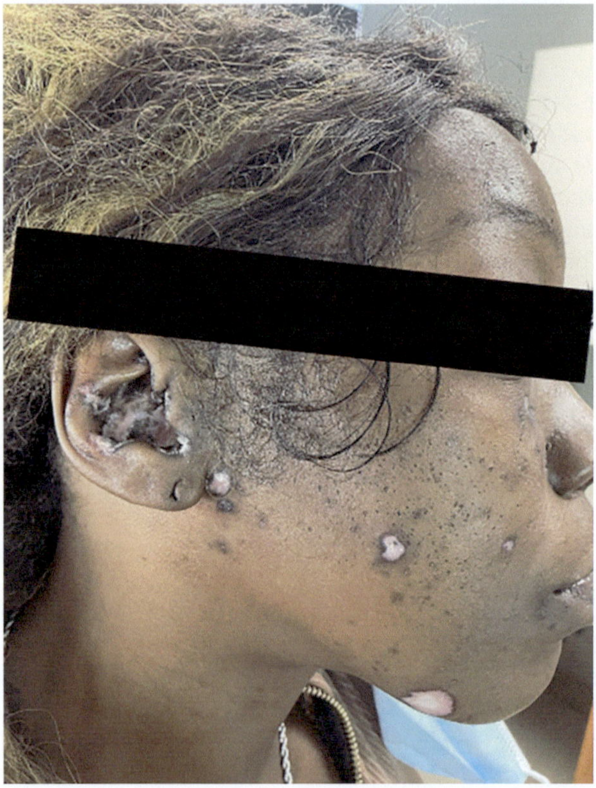

21. Cutaneous squamous cell carcinoma (SCC)

- Morphology/clinical features

  - Erythematous, scaly, papulonodule/plaque.

    - Some scale is thick and hyperkeratotic.

  - Squamous cell carcinoma in situ (Bowen's disease)—scaly, erythematous patch, or plaque.
  - Keratoacanthoma (SCC, KA type)—erythematous, hyperkeratotic doughnut-shaped papule with prominent central crust/ulceration.

- Verrucous carcinoma—various morphologies but includes epithelioma cuniculatum, Buschke–Lowenstein tumor, and oral florid papillomatosis.
  - Etiology is HPV-6 and HPV-11.

- Distribution
  - Commonly found on head/neck and dorsal extremities.
  - Epithelioma cuniculatum (seen on plantar foot), Buschke–Lowenstein tumor (seen in anogenital region), and oral florid papillomatosis (seen in oral cavity).

- Etiology/pathogenesis
  - Risk factors include chronic sun exposure, genetic syndromes, male gender, older age, fair skin, immunosuppression (i.e., transplant patients), HPV infection, radiation, long-standing nonhealing ulcers/wounds (Marjolin's ulcer), arsenic exposure, and chronic genital lichen sclerosus.

- Internal sequelae/comorbidities
  - Increased risk of systemic metastasis = immunosuppressed patient, location on lip/ear, diameter >2 cm, Breslow depth >2 mm, etiology is from burn/scar (Marjolin's ulcer), and poorly differentiated histology.

- Laboratory testing
  - Skin biopsy.

- Treatments/prognosis
  - Wide local excision, Mohs surgery, ED&C, and radiation therapy.

- USMLE Board Review Pearls
  - This is the second most common skin cancer with locally destructive effects as well as risk of metastasis and death. The risk of metastasis is much greater than basal cell carcinoma but still relatively low overall.
  - Sun exposure is the most common risk factor but other important ones include chemical carcinogens, radiation (occupational and therapeutic), chronic wounds (burn wounds), and immunosuppression (i.e., transplant patients).
  - Keratoacanthoma is a low-grade subtype of SCC.
  - A Marjolin ulcer is a rare type of SCC that develops in a chronic burn wound or ulcer, and it takes many years to form (like 5–10 years).
  - Multiple SCCs on the palmoplantar surface = arsenic exposure.
  - Bowen's disease on the penis is called erythroplasia of Queryat and presents as a solitary, velvety, erythematous plaque (patient will likely be elderly). Must biopsy to rule out Bowen's disease.
  - SCC on the lip has a high risk of metastasis and is more common on the lower lip.

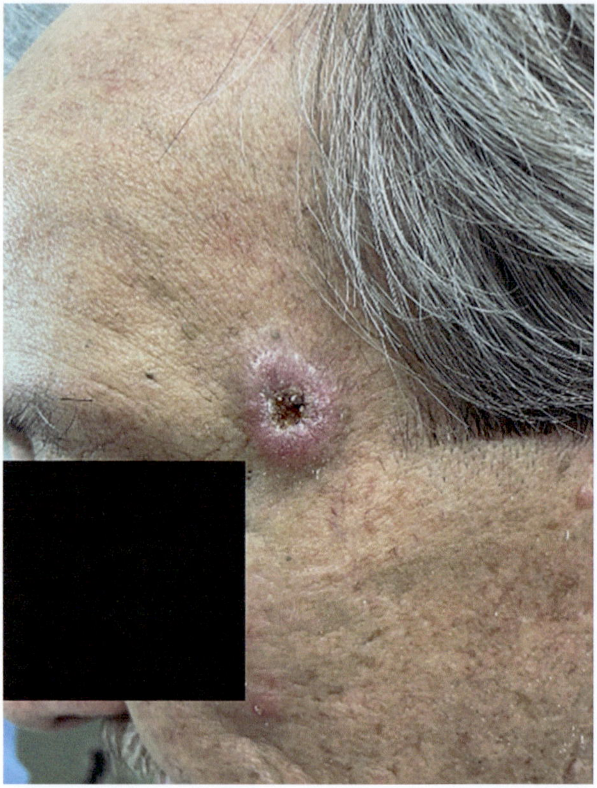

22. Darier disease

- Morphology/clinical features/distribution
  - Crusted, wart-like, red/brown papules and plaques on the head/neck and upper trunk.
    - Malodorous
  - Keratotic papules and pits on the palms.
  - Longitudinal red and white alternating nail streaks with distal notching in a "V" shape.
  - Oral cobblestoning in half of the affected patients.
  - Guttate leukoderma is a rarely described feature.
- Etiology/pathogenesis
  - Autosomal-dominant (AD) disorder due to a mutation in *ATP2A2*.
    - This mutation disturbs the calcium pump of the endoplasmic reticulum causing impaired synthesis of cell adhesion proteins.

- Internal sequelae/comorbidities
  - Increased incidence of epilepsy, intellectual impairment, bipolar disorder, and depression.
  - Prone to secondary infections.
- Laboratory testing
  - None.
- Treatments/prognosis
  - Difficult to treat but systemic retinoids are the treatment of choice.
- USMLE Board Review Pearls
  - Look for the characteristic skin/nail findings in a patient who is 13–20 years of age (peaks in puberty). The skin findings will be concentrated in a seborrheic distribution.
  - Due to a mutation in *ATP2A2*.
  - This is an AD disorder with complete penetrance and variable expressivity.
    - Patients can present with segmental disease as a result.
  - Kaposi's varicelliform eruption is the most worrisome secondary infection.

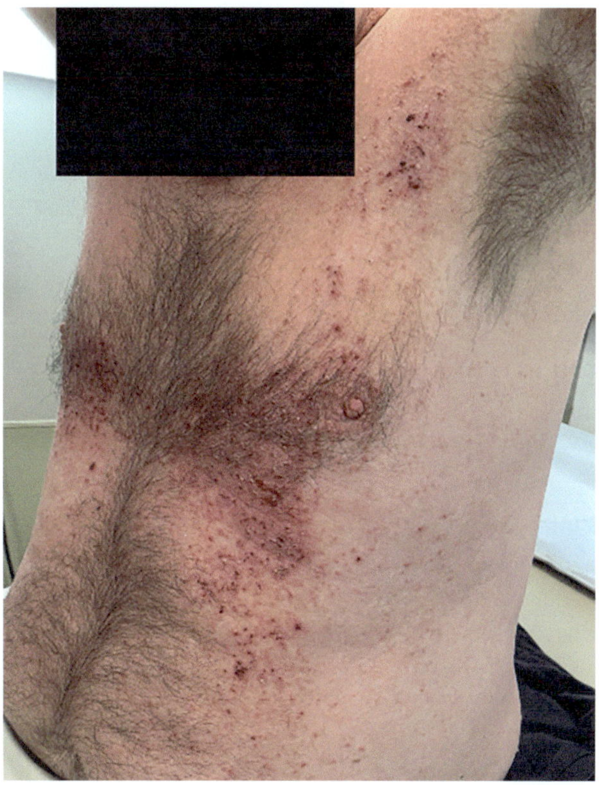

23. Delusions of parasitosis (DOP)

- Morphology/clinical features
  - Angulated and linear excoriations/erosions/ulcerations.
  - Patients may bring in "parasites" in a paper or plastic bag. This is called the matchbox sign.
  - There are different stages of delusions of parasitosis. Identifying them helps guide effective management. The "Koo-Brownstone Staging System" is the first and only staging system for patients who present with dermatological delusions. Please refer to the following article to review the staging and clinic features of DOP (*Brownstone N, Koo J. J Dermatolog Treat. 2022 Dec;33(8):3199-3201. doi: 10.1080/09546634.2022.2112548. Epub 2022 Aug 17*).
  - Patients present to the dermatologist because they believe they have a bona fide skin disease and often refuse to see a psychiatrist or mental health professional.
- Distribution
  - Commonly seen on the extremities and upper back (areas that the patient can reach with their fingers).
- Etiology/pathogenesis
  - This is a psychiatric disorder in which patients have delusions that they are infested with parasites or they see inanimate objects (such as fibers) coming of their skin.
- Internal sequelae/comorbidities
  - Must rule out secondary causes of delusions of parasitosis from alcohol or illicit drug use, organic brain injury, Axis I psychiatric disorders, hyperthyroidism, and vitamin B_{12} deficiency.
    - If a patient with schizophrenia presents with delusions of parasitosis, the diagnosis is schizophrenia and not delusions of parasitosis (i.e., the delusions of parasitosis is a psychotic feature of the patient's schizophrenia).
- Laboratory testing
  - None.
- Treatments/prognosis
  - First must rule out any bona fide skin diseases (such as scabies infestation).
  - Treatment of choice is pimozide in primary cases (a first-generation neuroleptic) because this medication has no FDA-approved indication for any psychiatric disorders (it is only FDA approved for Tourette syndrome, which is a neurological disease), so patients with DOP will be amenable to taking it.

  - Second-generation antipsychotics work well but patients with DOP are reluctant to take them because they do not believe they have a psychiatric disorder.
  - The most important goal is to establish a rapport with the patient before offering therapy!

- USMLE Board Review Pearls

  - Delusional disorder is a fixed, false belief and can be nonbizarre ("The CIA is tracking me") or bizarre ("I am an Alien from Outer Space").

    - Subtypes include jealous, paranoid, somatic (DOP is under this subtype), erotomaniac, and grandiose.
    - Symptoms must be present > 1 month and day-to-day functioning is mostly unaffected.
    - *Folie à deux:* a shared delusion between two people—treatment of choice is to separate the patients and treat individually.

      - This is sometimes seen with DOP patients.

  - Treatment of choice is pimozide for DOP and must rule out secondary causes of DOP (in that case the treatment of choice is to treat underlying disorder such as schizophrenia).

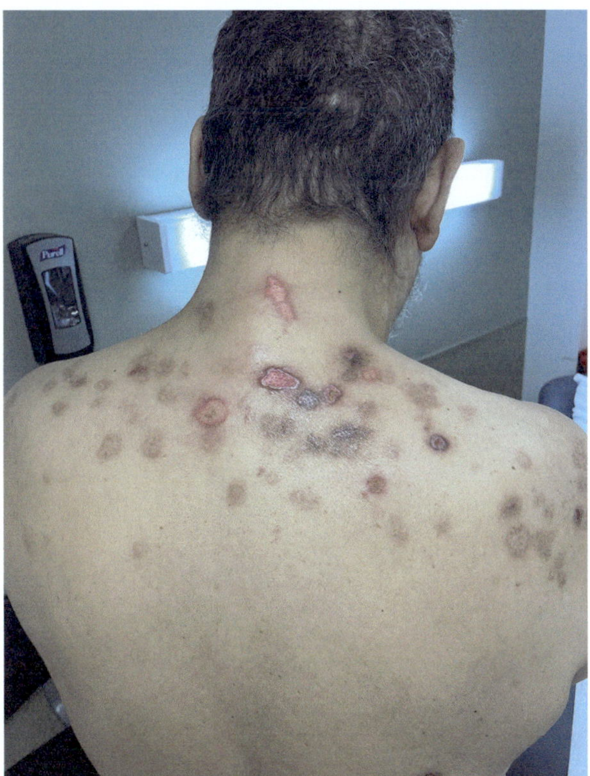

24. Dermatitis herpetiformis (DH)

- Morphology/clinical features
  - VERY ITCHY herpetiform and fragile vesicles on an urticarial base.
    - The pruritus is usually so severe that patients just present with excoriated papules/erosions because the fragile vesicles have been scratched off.
- Distribution
  - Classily seen on extensor extremities, buttocks, and back/neck.
  - Less commonly seen on the face/scalp including the nose.
- Etiology/pathogenesis
  - Gluten is a grain protein (found mainly in wheat, rye, and barley) and gliadin is the antigenic component of gluten, and once ingested the gliadin is modified by the lamina propria (transglutaminase protein present in GI lamina propria [TTG2]-gliadin neoantigen), causing the formation of antibodies. Due to epitope spreading, IgA autoantibodies target TTG3 (epidermal transglutaminase) in the skin, causing inflammation and blisters due to cell damage.
- Internal sequelae/comorbidities
  - Strongly associated with autoimmune diseases.
    - Hashimoto's thyroiditis (most common), diabetes mellitus, and pernicious anemia.
    - Less commonly associated with Addison's disease, alopecia areata, myasthenia gravis, vitiligo, and systemic lupus.
  - Only 20% of patients with DH have symptomatic GI disease, but nearly all have some degree of gluten-sensitive enteropathy on GI biopsy.
    - Therefore, do not ask a patient with suspected DH if they have any GI issues, they will likely say no.
- Laboratory testing
  - Antiendomysial antibodies
    - Titers correlate with degree of gluten-related enteropathy.
  - Tissue transglutaminase-2 (tTG- IgA)
    - Highly sensitive and specific
    - Marker of GI involvement
- Treatments/prognosis
  - A gluten-free diet treats both the skin disease and GI disease.
    - This is the only therapy that decreases the risk of GI lymphoma.

- Treatment of choice for the skin disease and pruritus is dapsone.
  - Controls the symptoms in 2–3 days.
  - Don't forget to check for G6PD deficiency before initiating dapsone.

- USMLE Board Review Pearls
  - Look for symmetric, bilateral, pruritic papules, vesicles, bullae, and erosions on the elbows, knees, buttocks, neck, and scalp in a patient who is 30–40 years old.
  - Associated with celiac disease
    - This can be thought of as the skin manifestation of celiac disease.
  - Treatment of choice is gluten-free diet and dapsone.
  - This disease has nothing to do with herpes simplex virus, despite the name herpetiformis.
  - Patients must stick to a CROP diet (corn, rice, oats, and potatoes).
  - NSAIDs, seaweed, and iodine classically exacerbate DH.
  - This is the only known disease in dermatology where the split is in the lamina lucida of the basement membrane but the antibodies are found in the papillary dermis.

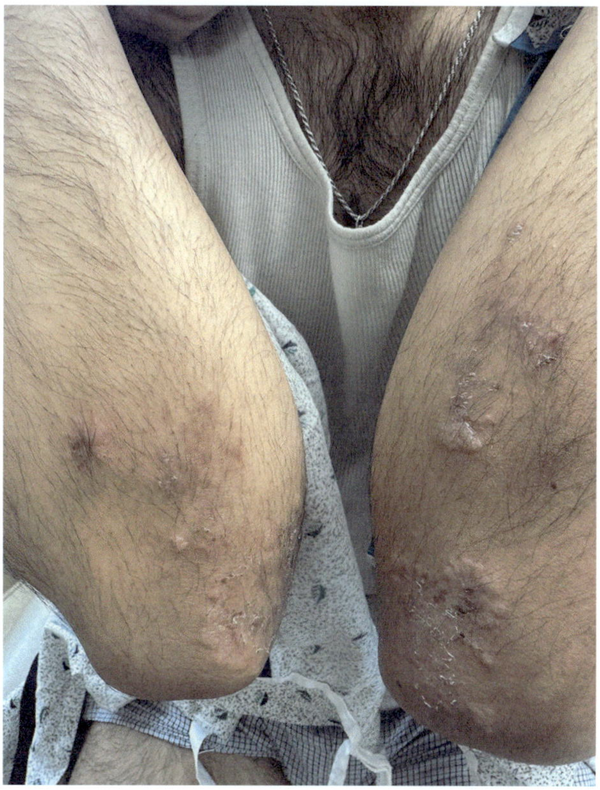

25. Dermatofibroma (DF)/Dermatofibrosarcoma Protuberans (DFSP)

- Morphology/clinical features
  - DF—**firm** dermal papule with overlying hyperpigmentation.
    - "Dimple sign"—moves downward when the adjacent skin is pinched together.
    - Benign skin lesion.
  - DFSP—firm expanding plaque with multinodular morphology.
    - "Nodules in a plaque."
    - Slow-growing malignancy.
- Distribution
  - DFs are commonly seen on the extremities.
  - DSFPs favor trunk (shoulder number 1), proximal extremities.
    - Less commonly on the head/neck.
- Etiology/pathogenesis
  - DF—unknown but associated with previous bug bites and trauma.
  - DFSP—malignancy characterized by t(17;22) COL1A1-PDGFB fusion gene.
- Internal sequelae/comorbidities
  - DF—none.
    - Multiple eruptive DFs can be associated with HIV or lupus.
  - DFSP—very low risk of metastatic potential (< 1%).
- Laboratory testing
  - None.
- Treatments/prognosis
  - DF—can surgically excise for cosmetic reasons.
  - DFSP—treatment of choice is Mohs surgery.
    - Can also do WLE with 2–3 cm down to fascia.
    - Imatinib is approved for unresectable or metastatic disease.
- USMLE Board Review Pearls
  - DF—look for dome-shaped, firm, brown-pink, nontender nodule that dimples when pinched; treatment is optional.
  - DFSP—look for a hyperpigmented/brown plaque with multinodular appearance; treatment of choice is Mohs surgery.
  - DF is a benign lesion and DFSP is a malignancy.
  - DFSP stains with CD34.

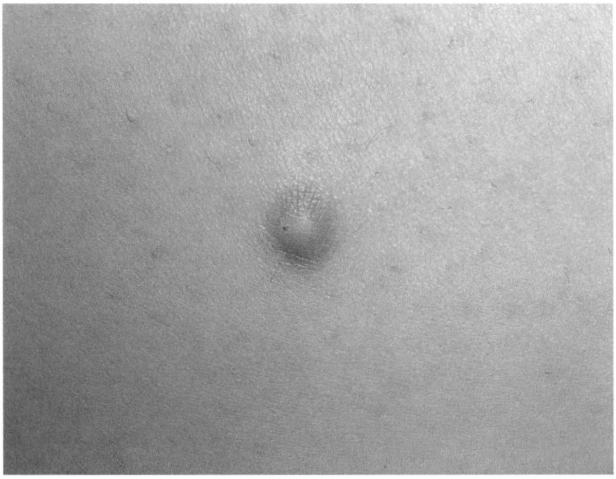

26. Dermatomyositis (DM)

- Morphology/clinical features/distribution
  - Symmetric, proximal muscle weakness (extensors > flexors) **without** muscle pain.
- Shoulder, hip girdle, and neck flexor weakness manifested by difficulty walking upstairs, standing from sitting position, brushing hair.
  - Gottron's papules = lichenoid, pink/erythematous papules, overlying the hand joints
    - Gottron's sign = macular erythema overlying the hand joints, elbows, knees, DIP, PIP, and MCP joints.
  - Symmetric confluent macular violaceous erythema = facial/malar erythema classically involving the melolabial folds (vs. ACLE, which spares the nasolabial fold).
  - Heliotrope sign = periorbital edema and erythema on the eyelids.
    - Due to inflammation of the orbicularis oculi muscle.
  - Holster and shawl/V- sign = erythematous/violaceous macular patches over the lateral thigh and upper back/chest, respectively.
  - Nail changes include "ragged" cuticles and proximal nailfolds with dilated capillary loops alternating with areas of vessel dropout.
- Etiology/pathogenesis
  - Exact pathogenesis unknown; this is theorized to be caused by environmental/external factors (such as malignancy or infection), triggering an immune-mediated autoimmune reaction in patients with a genetic susceptibility.
  - Drug-induced DM

  - Hydroxyurea (50% of cases but this drug is rarely used anymore), statins, D-penicillamine, and cyclophosphamide.

- Internal sequelae/comorbidities
  - Adult DM
    - Malignancy (ovarian, GI, nasopharyngeal carcinoma in Asians), breast, lung, pancreatic, and non-Hodgkin's lymphoma.
    - Can present before diagnosis, at the time of diagnosis or after diagnosis.
      - Most are detected 1–2 years within diagnosis and risk returns to baseline 5 years after diagnosis (except for GI cancers and pancreatic cancer).
  - Anti-synthetase syndrome
    - Rapid onset of disease a/w constitutional symptoms, Raynaud's, mechanics hands (hyperkeratosis and scaling), nonerosive arthritis, and interstitial lung disease.
  - Anti-CADM-140 (MDA5) antibodies in DM.
    - a/w interstitial lung disease.
  - Juvenile DM
    - There is no increased risk of cancer!
    - A/w intussusception and calcinosis cutis.
- Laboratory testing
  - ANA, CPK, and aldolase.
  - Muscle biopsy is gold standard.
- Treatments/prognosis
  - Skin limited disease
    - Photoprotection, topical corticosteroids.
    - Recheck muscle enzyme every 2–3 months to monitor for muscle involvement; if positive, treat with systemic medications.
  - Skin + muscle disease
    - PO prednisone and add methotrexate if patient is not responding.
    - Can do IVIG as a steroid-sparing option.
- USMLE Board Review Pearls
  - Look for the classic skin rash (heliotrope sign, "shawl sign," Gottron's papules) in a patient with muscle weakness.
    - Either heliotrope sign and Gottron's papules are almost always shown on exams.

- Gottron's papules = papules with scale on the dorsum of the hand OVERLYING the joints.
- The biopsy of DM shows subtle vacuolar interface dermatitis, epidermal atrophy and peri- adnexal and perivascular inflammation with considerable interstitial mucin deposition.
- Dermatomyositis can be associated with occult malignancy.
- Antibodies that are associated with DM.
  - Anti-Jo-1 (histidyl-tRNA synthetase) = anti-synthetase syndrome.
  - Anti-SRP (signal recognition particle) = acute-onset necrotizing myopathy, may be refractory to treatment.
  - Anti-Mi-2 (helicase) = **good prognosis** and classic skin findings in DM.
  - Anti-TIF-1γ (p155) = high risk of malignancy. Anti-NXP-2 (p140) = high risk of malignancy, a/w calcinosis.
    - Patients cannot have more than one myositis antibody.
- 1/3 of patients with DM who take hydroxychloroquine will get a morbilliform drug eruption.

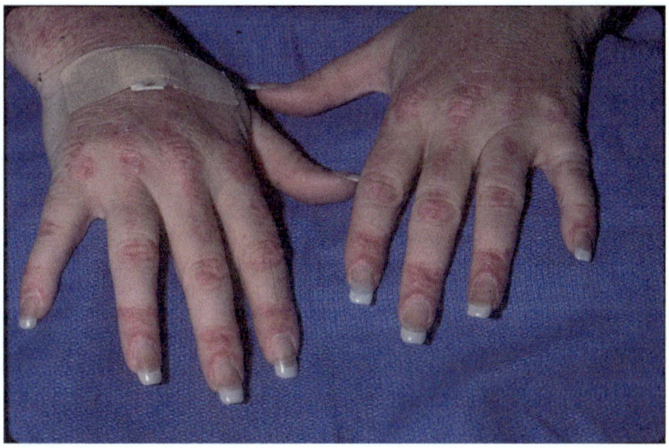

27. Drug eruptions

- Morphology/clinical features/distribution.
- Drug eruptions are sometimes difficult to diagnosis clinically because there can be many overlapping features and the dermatopathology usually does not help in easily differentiating between different drug eruptions. **The most important diagnostic pearl in the evaluation of a drug rash patient is to determine the most likely culprit agent and the timeline** (i.e., how soon after the suspected culprit drug was started did the eruption develop?). There are then some clinical features that will help in distinguishing between drug eruptions and arriving at a definitive diagnosis (such as the acute onset of bullae in SJS/TEN or prominent facial erythema/edema in DRESS).
  - Morbilliform drug (MDE)—symmetrically distributed erythematous macules, papules, and/or urticarial lesions that start on the trunk /extremi-

ties and may become confluent over time. Areas may even appear as atypical targetoid lesions, leading to the misdiagnosis of erythema multiforme.

  - **Typical time course 4–14 days but as early as 2 days in rechallenge.**

- Drug Reaction with Eosinophilia and Systemic Systems (DRESS)—fever and cutaneous eruption appearing as morbilliform in nature starting on the face, upper trunk, and extremities, which becomes edematous and extensive. Patients with DRESS look sick and feel sick as opposed to patients with morbilliform drug eruption. **Edema/erythema of the face is a common finding.**

  - **Typical time course 2–8 weeks.**

- Acute generalized exanthematous pustulosis (AGEP)—fever and numerous small, pinpoint, sterile pustules arise within large plaques of edematous erythema initially appearing on the face and skin folds.

  - **Typical time course 1–4 days.**

- Stevens–Johnson syndrome/toxic epidermal necrolysis (SJS/TEN)—lesions appear as erythematous, dusky red, or purpuric macules of irregular size and shape, which coalesce, leading to acute bullae and skin necrosis associated with skin pain, fever, painful eyes, pain upon swallowing/micturition, and erosions/erythema of the mucosal membranes, including ocular, genital, and oral.

  - SJS: <10% of body surface area (BSA).
  - TEN: >30% of BSA.

    - **Typical time course initial week(s) of therapy to months.**
    - **For aromatic anticonvulsants, the risk is greatest during the first two months of treatment.**

- Fixed drug eruption (FDE)/bullous FDE—one or more round to oval, sharply demarcated, erythematous to dusky violet plaques that can appear anywhere on the body. Bullous FDE is FDE with bullae and can become quite extensive. Mucosal membranes may be involved. Upon rechallenge, the lesions will appear in the exact same spot as before with a possibility of new spots forming.

  - **Typical time course 2–14 days but as early as 24 hours in rechallenge.**

- Progressive immunotherapy-related mucocutaneous eruption (PIRME)—a newly described drug reaction that mimics SJS/TEN both clinically and histologically that is due to immune checkpoint inhibitors (such as pembrolizumab or atezolizumab). It has a benign course and usually has a delayed onset. Since these medications are life-saving cancer therapies, the recognition of PIRME is important because patients can keep receiving the drug as opposed to a diagnosis of SJS/TEN.

- Most common drug triggers
  - MDE—most drugs can cause this but high-risk ones include aminopenicillins, allopurinol, sulfonamides, cephalosporins, and anticonvulsants.
  - DRESS—aromatic anticonvulsants, lamotrigine, sulfonamides, vancomycin, minocycline, allopurinol, dapsone, HIV medications (e.g., abacavir), and targeted therapies for cancer (e.g., vemurafenib).
  - AGEP—antibiotics (aminopenicillins, cephalosporins, clindamycin) and calcium channel blockers.
  - SJS/TEN—allopurinol, antibiotics, nonsteroidal anti-inflammatory drugs, and aromatic anticonvulsants.
  - FDE—antibiotics (sulfonamides, tetracyclines > β-lactams, fluoroquinolones, macrolides), NSAIDs, acetaminophen, aspirin, barbiturates, dapsone, proton pump inhibitors, and azole antifungals.
- Internal sequelae/comorbidities
  - MDE—none.
  - DRESS—most commonly fever, lymphadenopathy and eosinophilia. Patients may also develop renal involvement (e.g., interstitial nephritis), myocarditis, interstitial pneumonitis, myositis, and thyroiditis.
    - Eosinophilia may be delayed by up to 2 weeks and is commonly not present when DRESS is due to lamotrigine.
  - AGEP—none.
  - SJS/TEN—death from infection and fluid loss. Survivors may develop symblepharon, conjunctival synechiae, entropion, ingrowth of eyelashes, scarring, dyspigmentation, eruptive melanocytic nevi, urethral stenosis, phimosis, nail dystrophy, hair loss, dry eyes, and even blindness.
  - FDE—none.
- Laboratory testing
  - DRESS—CBC, LFTs.
- Treatments/prognosis
  - MDE—supportive care, can continue the drug if necessary.
  - DRESS—**stop the drug!** slow taper of PO steroids over 3–6 months, and mortality rate ranges from 2 to 10%.
  - AGEP—supportive care, PO steroids for pruritus.
  - SJS/TEN—**stop the drug!** IVIG, etanercept, systemic steroids, cyclosporine, and mortality rate ranges from 5 to 20%.
  - FDE—supportive care.
  - PIRME—supportive care, patients eventually may continue receiving the drug.

- USMLE Board Review Pearls
  - Always think of a drug reaction in any hospitalized patient who develops an acute cutaneous eruption!
  - A common site for FDE is the penis.
    - In the appropriate clinical context, this diagnosis should always be considered for any acute eruption involving the penis.
  - Another name for DRESS is DIHS, which stands for drug-induced hypersensitivity syndrome.
  - Look for these common medications as a cause of DRESS on exams: phenytoin, carbamazepine, minocycline, sulfa drugs, allopurinol, and vancomycin.
  - Look for these common medications as a cause of SJS/TEN on exams: sulfonamides, seizure medications (phenytoin, carbamazepine, lamotrigine), quinolones, and antiretroviral drugs (especially NNRTIs).
  - TEN involves greater than 30% BSA and skin lesions may initially appear targetoid as in erythema multiforme. Mucosal involvement is present in nearly all cases (which includes eyes, mouth, and genitals).
  - The most important initial step in treating any DRESS or SJS/TEN patient is to immediately stop the culprit drug and ensure it is not given ever again.
  - Supportive care for patients with morbilliform drug eruptions includes antihistamines and topical corticosteroids.
  - Treatment of SJS/TEN may include systemic steroids, etanercept, IVIG, and cyclosporine.
  - A biopsy of SJS/TEN will show full-thickness epidermal necrosis without significant inflammation.
  - SJS/TEN patients should ideally be treated as burn victims in the burn ICU with specific management of thermoregulation, electrolyte disturbances, secondary infections, and dressing changes.

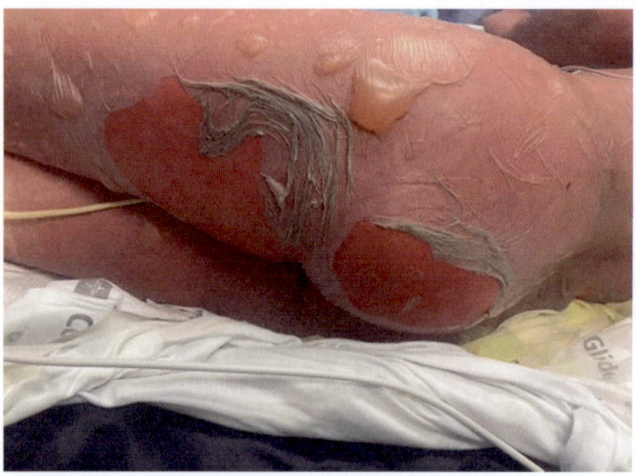

28. Erythema annulare centrifugum (EAC)

- Morphology/clinical features
  - Annular/polycyclic plaques that migrate centrifugally that start as macules with characteristic "trailing scale" (trailing scale is a circular fine line of scaling that is just inside the area of erythema, i.e., it is lagging or "trailing" behind the spreading rash).
  - Can migrate as much as 2–12 mm in 12 hours.
  - Usually not pruritic.
  - The herald patch of pityriasis rosea resembles EAC both clinically and histologically.
- Distribution
  - Commonly seen on the trunk, axilla, and proximal extremities.
- Etiology/pathogenesis
  - Unknown but thought to be an immune reaction to an infection.
    - The most common association is with tinea (dermatophyte) infection.
  - Diagnosis of exclusion; this condition is overdiagnosed!
    - Must rule out tinea (dermatophyte infection), pityriasis rosea, eczema, and resolving pustular psoriasis.
  - Peaks in the fifth decade of life.
- Internal sequelae/comorbidities
  - None.
  - Some sources state that it is secondary to neoplasms (usually lymphoproliferative malignancies).
- Laboratory testing
  - None.
- Treatments/prognosis
  - Treat underlying disorder.
  - Topical steroids if symptomatic.
  - Lesions will likely resolve on their own but may last months.
- USMLE Board Review Pearls
  - Look for the characteristic eruption in a patient with a history of an infection (most commonly a dermatophyte infection like tinea pedis).
  - Most commonly seen on hips/thighs.
  - The patient will notice that the rash is expanding.
  - Do not confuse with erythema migrans, which is nonscaly.

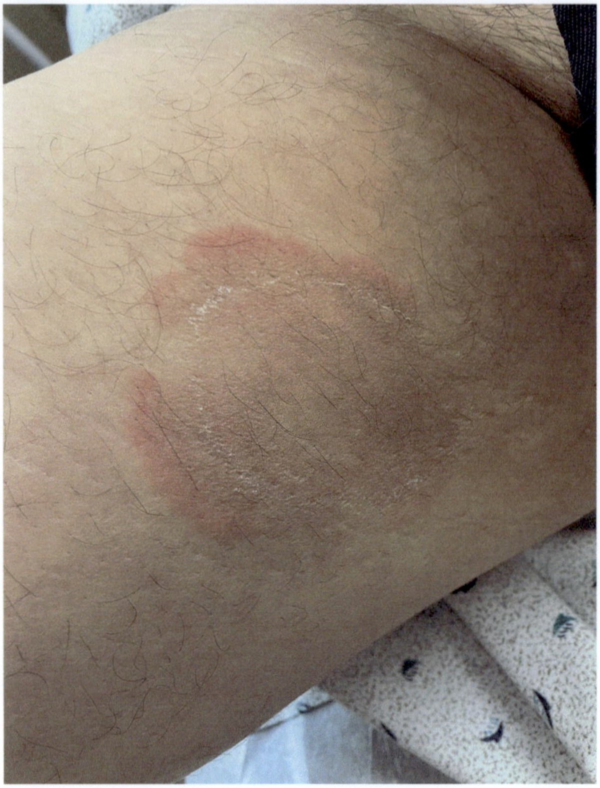

29. Eosinophilic fasciitis (Shulman syndrome)

- Morphology/clinical features
  - Rapid onset of symmetric edematous/indurated areas of skin that progresses to peau d'orange ("pseudeo-cellulite") and woody appearing plaques.
  - "Dry river bed" sign = linear depressions of veins within the background of indurated and tightly bound skin.
- Distribution
  - Extremities
    - Can rarely be seen on the trunk.
- Etiology/pathogenesis
  - Classically associated with recent history of strenuous activity such as marathon running or intense weightlifting.
    - Other reported causes include trauma, borreliosis, and statin use.
  - Unknown but thought to be related to large increase in TGF-β.

- Internal sequelae/comorbidities
  - No internal comorbidities.
  - Joint contractures may develop.
- Laboratory testing
  - CBC with diff.
    - Peripheral eosinophilia seen in nearly all cases.
  - MRI will show thickened fascia.
- Treatments/prognosis
  - PO prednisone.
  - Steroid-staring therapies: methotrexate, acitretin, and TNF-α inhibitors.
  - Physical therapy for joint contractures.
  - Up to 1/3 of cases may resolve spontaneously; however, residual induration may be present.
  - IL-6 inhibitors (i.e., tocilizumab) have been recently described as successful in steroid-refractory cases.
- USMLE Board Review Pearls
  - Look for indurated, rippled, "orange-peel"-appearing plaques on the extremities in a patient with recent history of intense physical activity like training for a marathon or power-lifting.
  - Tissue eosinophilia is not essential for diagnosis but should see peripheral eosinophilia.
  - Lacks prominent systemic symptoms.
  - Treatment of choice is systemic steroids and disease response should be appreciated as soon as 2–3 weeks.

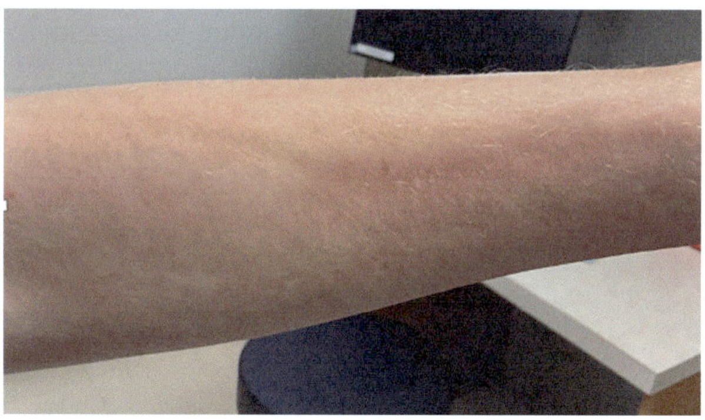

30. Erosive pustular dermatosis

- Morphology/clinical features
  - Pustules, crusts, and erosions.
    - Patient will likely be older and photodamaged.
- Distribution
  - Scalp.
  - Rarely can be seen on lower extremities in the setting of venous insufficiency.
- Etiology/pathogenesis
  - Unknown but etiologies include trauma, medications, comorbid conditions, and history of several dermatological procedures to the affected area.
- Internal sequelae/comorbidities
  - Possibly a/w autoimmune thyroiditis.
- Laboratory testing
  - None.
- Treatments/prognosis
  - Topical corticosteroids and topical calcineurin inhibitors.
- USMLE Board Review Pearls
  - This is often confused for SCC of the scalp.
    - The biopsy features will be nonspecific, and if there is no evidence of SCC, then the diagnosis is erosive pustular dermatosis.
  - Mainly a disease of the elderly that is due to sun damage and multiple procedures such as repeated rounds of cryosurgery for actinic keratoses.

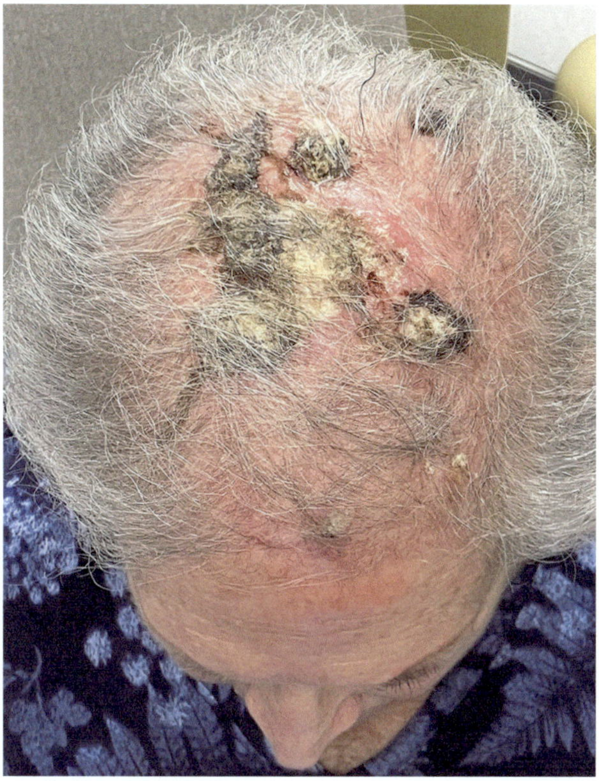

31. Erysipelas

- Morphology/clinical features
  - Sharply defined plaque with "fiery-red" color with "ridge-like" borders.
    - a/w pain and burning.
- Distribution
  - Lower extremity is the most common site.
  - Can also be seen on the face.
- Etiology/pathogenesis
  - Group A β-hemolytic *strep*.
  - More superficial variant of cellulitis that involves the upper-mid dermis.
    - Cellulitis is a deeper infection.
- Internal sequelae/comorbidities
  - Lymphedema is an important risk factor.

- Laboratory testing
  - Increased DNase B and ASO titers.
  - Wound/blood cultures usually negative.
- Treatments/prognosis
  - Penicillin for 10–14 days.
    - Erythromycin if penicillin allergy.
- USMLE Board Review Pearls
  - Look for a well-defined, raised, tender, and edematous plaque between normal and infected skin.
    - Patient may have fever or chills.
  - This is an infection involving the upper dermis and lymphatic channels.
  - Group A *strep* is the most commonly implicated bacteria, and penicillin is the treatment of choice.
  - In children, it can present as a small red patch on the cheek or extremities that rapidly turns into the characteristic red plaque.
  - Do not confuse with ecthyma, which is also caused by *strep*.

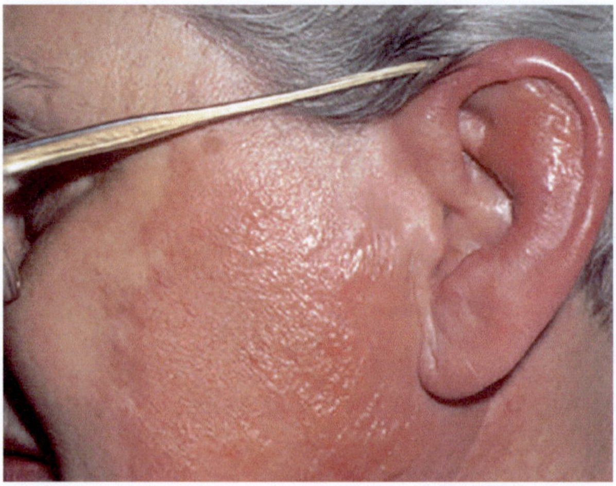

32. Erythema ab igne

- Morphology/clinical features
  - Thick, reticulated erythema or post-inflammatory hyperpigmentation in a net-like pattern.

- Distribution
  - Shins, lower back, knees, and anterior thighs.
- Etiology/pathogenesis
  - Chronic, repeated, nonburning, heat, or infrared radiation exposure to a well-defined anatomical site.
  - Shins
    - Usually due to space heaters.
  - Lower back/knees
    - Usually due to heating pads.
  - Anterior thighs
    - Usually due to laptops.
- Internal sequelae/comorbidities
  - Possible increased risk of SCC
    - Latent period is long, nearly 30 years, and highest risk with hydrocarbon-fueled heat exposure.
    - Relatively no concern for SCC from household exposures.
- Laboratory testing
  - None.
- Treatments/prognosis
  - Counsel patient on etiology and to stop the heat source.
  - Workup underlying cause of pain that is necessitating the heating pad, if appropriate.
- USMLE Board Review Pearls
  - Look for a patient with a history of back pain or knee pain who constantly uses a heating pad.
    - The patient will likely have had surgery in the area and a surgical scar may be visible.
  - Treatment of choice is counseling the patient on the etiology and stopping the heat source to the area.
  - Most commonly seen in the lumbosacral region.

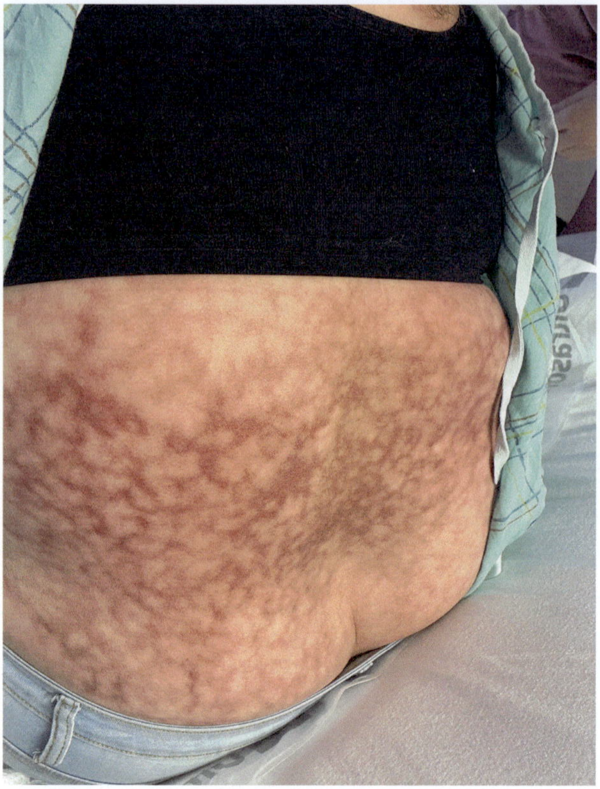

33. Erythema dyschromicum perstans (EDP)
    - Morphology/clinical features
      - Slate gray/blue oval macules coalescing into patches.
        - Sometimes these patches can have an erythematous rim.
      - Asymptomatic.
      - Also referred to as "ashy dermatosis" due to the characteristic color.
    - Distribution
      - Symmetric eruption of upper trunk, neck, and extremities.
    - Etiology/pathogenesis
      - Unknown but theorized to be secondary to pollutants in the environment causing disease in predisposed individuals.
    - Internal sequelae/comorbidities
      - None.

- Laboratory testing
  - None.
- Treatments/prognosis
  - Difficult to treat effectively!
  - Clofazimine is the treatment choice, but this medication is rarely used in clinical practice and the efficacy is questionable.
  - A systematic review demonstrated that NB-UVB was effective.
  - A small case series demonstrated efficacy of prednisone and isotretinoin in the early inflammatory phase of disease.
- USMLE Board Review Pearls
  - Histology mimics post-inflammatory hyperpigmentation, and the direct immunofluorescence pattern mimics lichen planus.
  - Most pediatric cases will resolve spontaneously within a few years, but in adults the disease is more persistent.
  - These patients are asymptomatic.

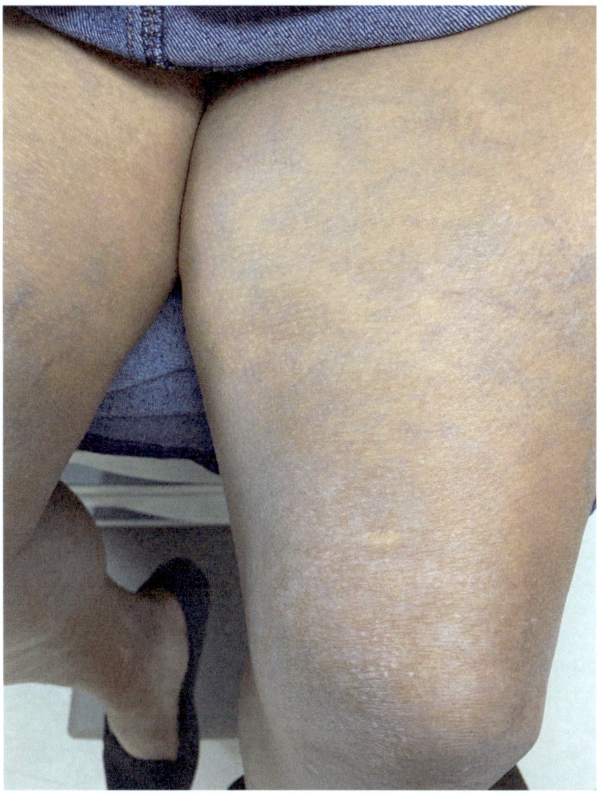

34. Erythema migrans

- Morphology/clinical features
  - Annular, red, round to oval expanding patch.
    - Sometimes resembles a "bull's eye" with a light-colored central area.
    - Usually less than 5 cm in diameter.
    - Center may become dark, violaceus, or vesicular.
    - Multiple smaller similar rashes can be seen due to disseminated disease.
  - Asymptomatic!
- Distribution
  - Trunk and intertriginous areas (axilla, groin, and popliteal fossa).
  - The patches usually follow skin lines.
- Etiology/pathogenesis
  - Due to *Borrelia burgdorferi* (a spirochete).
- Internal sequelae/comorbidities
  - If untreated can lead to Lyme disease.
    - Early localized disease = flu-like symptoms and lymphadenopathy.
    - Early disseminated disease = Bell's palsy, arthralgias, heart block, iritis.
    - Chronic disease = chronic monoarticular arthritis (large joints), encephalopathy, acrodermatitis chronica atrophicans (in Europe).
- Laboratory testing
  - ELISA test for anti-*Borrelia burgdorferi* antibodies.
    - Peak IgM response occurs 3–6 weeks after infection, so only about 25% of patients will have a positive test during acute phase of infection.
- Treatments/prognosis
  - Doxycycline 100 mg BID for 14 days.
  - Amoxicillin 16 mg/kg TID for 14 days (children < 8 years old).
    - Amoxicillin is preferred but the American Academy of Pediatrics considers use of doxycycline for ≤21 days to be acceptable in children <8 years of age.
  - If you miss this diagnosis, then the rash will go away, but the patient will be at risk of progressing to Lyme disease.

- USMLE Board Review Pearls
  - Lyme disease is an infection caused by *Borrelia burgdorferi* that usually peaks during the summer months and the vector is the *Ixodes* tick, which is found on white-tailed deer and white-footed mice.
    - Endemic to the Northeast, Northern Midwest, and Pacific Coast.
  - Infection usually occurs after the tick has been feeding on the skin for > 36 hours.
  - Look for a "bull's-eye" or oval/round erythematous patch in a patient who presents during the summer months from the Northeastern part of the United States.
    - Be especially suspicious if the patient reports recently hiking or camping.
  - Secondary or early disseminated Lyme disease presents with migratory polyarthritis, neurologic disease (facial nerve palsy, b/l is classic), meningitis, myocarditis, and third-degree AV block.
  - Tertiary (late disease)—arthritis and subacute encephalitis (manifested by memory loss and mood change).
  - Early disease is diagnosed by clinical presentation alone! (erythema migrans + endemic area). Later stages can be diagnosed with serology. If IgM or IgG ELISA is positive, then confirm with Western blot.
  - Must remove tick if visible on skin exam gently with forceps. Don't forget to disinfect the area. Treat early disease with PO doxycycline. More advanced disease requires IV ceftriaxone.
  - Prophylaxis = one dose of PO doxycycline if all of the following apply:
    - Identified *Ixodes* tick that has been attached for >36 hours.
    - Prophylaxis is started <72 hours after removal.
    - Patient has no contraindications to PO doxy and local rate of infection of ticks with *Borrelia* is >20%.
      - If the above criteria are not met, then observe and treat only if erythema migrans subsequently develops.

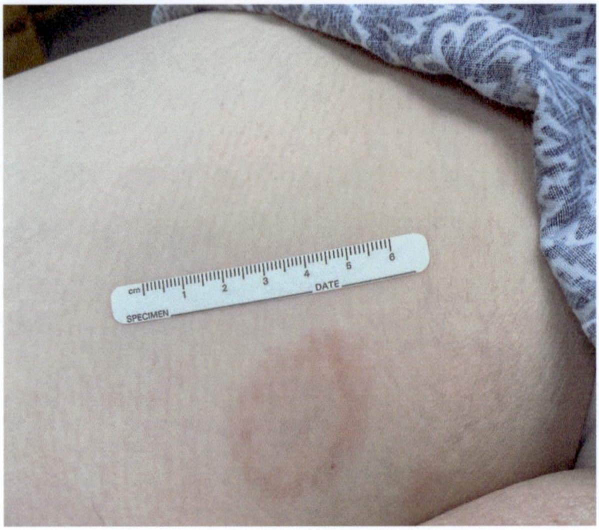

35. Erythema multiforme (EM)

- Morphology/clinical features
  - Symmetric, fixed, red macules and papules that develop into "target" lesions.
    - A typical target has three zones.
      - Dusky or necrotic center, edematous pale surrounding ring, and outer rim of erythema.
  - EM minor
    - Target lesions with minimal mucosal involvement and no systemic symptoms.
  - EM major
    - Target lesions with severe mucosal involvement and systemic symptoms (fever and joint pain).
  - This disease is often overdiagnosed! Targetoid lesions do not automatically mean a diagnosis of EM. Must rule out other skin diseases that may present with a targetoid-like appearance.

- Distribution
  - Acrofacial
    - Favors oral mucosa and b/l distal extremities, including palms and soles.
- Etiology/pathogenesis
  - Nearly all cases caused by infection, and the most common trigger is HSV.
  - Others include *Mycoplasma pneumoniae* and *Histoplasma capsulatum* (can see with concomitant erythema nodosum).
- Internal sequelae/comorbidities
  - None.
- Laboratory testing
  - 80% of patients have detectable HSV by PCR in the early stages in the target lesions.
- Treatments/prognosis
  - Symptomatic treatment.
  - HSV prophylaxis to prevent future outbreaks if appropriate.
- USMLE Board Review Pearls
  - Herpes simplex is the most common cause.
    - Another common infectious trigger is *Mycoplasma pneumoniae.*
  - Look for the classic targetoid lesions on the palms, soles, and crusting/erosions on the lips. Patients may have systemic symptoms such as fever, myalgias, arthralgias, and headaches.
  - Nikolsky sign is negative, and there is no risk of progression to TEN.
  - Drug triggers of EM include sulfa drugs, β-lactams, and antiepileptics, but this is an uncommon cause.

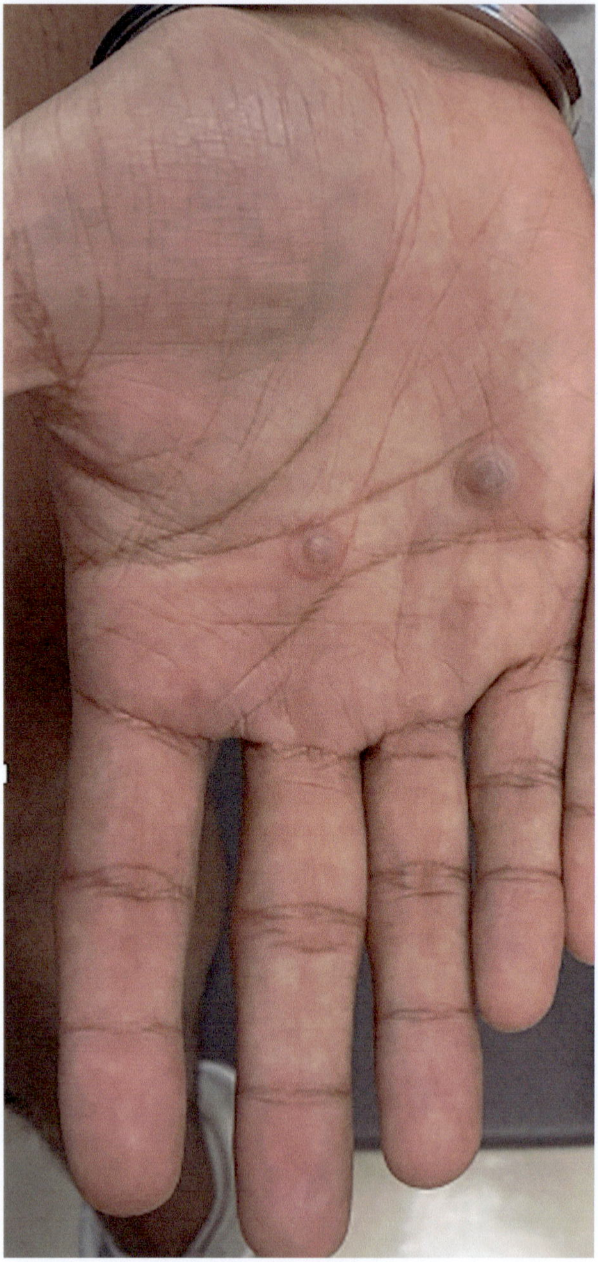

36. Erythema nodosum

- Morphology/clinical features
  - Acute, tender, subcutaneous nodules with overlying erythema or bruise-like patches.
  - This is the most common panniculitis.
- Distribution
  - Pretibial areas.
- Etiology/pathogenesis
  - Delayed hypersensitivity response to various antigens (Th1 axis).
  - Most common cause is idiopathic.
  - Infections
    - *Strep* infections (most common cause), other infections (bacterial GI infections [*Yersinia, Salmonella, Campylobacter*], viral URIs, coccidioidomycosis, TB, and histoplasmosis).
  - Drugs
    - Estrogens/OCPs, sulfa drugs, and NSAIDs.
- Internal sequelae/comorbidities
  - A/w sarcoidosis and inflammatory bowel disease.
- Laboratory testing
  - None.
- Treatments/prognosis
  - Develops acutely over 1–2 weeks, then resolves spontaneously.
    - New lesions may develop over a few months duration.
  - Treat underlying issues if identifiable.
  - Symptomatic treatment and supportive care.
- USMLE Board Review Pearls
  - Look for painful and erythematous nodules on the anterior shins that slowly progress and appear bruised in later stages without ulceration.
  - This disease is a form of panniculitis (inflammation of the subcutaneous adipose tissue).
  - Causes include *strep* infection, coccidioides, *Yersinia pestis*, TB, sulfa drugs, antibiotics, oral contraceptive pills, sarcoidosis, Crohn's disease, ulcerative colitis, and Behçet disease/leprosy (rare).

- Due to these causes, a general workup should include ASO titer, PPD (in high-risk patients), CXR, and GI consult to rule out inflammatory bowel disease.
- Causes can be remembered with the mnemonic NODOSUMS
  - **NO** cause (idiopathic)
  - **D**rugs
  - **O**ral contraceptives
  - **S**arcoidosis
  - **U**lcerative colitis/Crohn's disease
  - **M**icrobiology (various infections)
  - ***S****trep* (number 1 infectious cause)

– Treatment includes cool compresses, bed rest, elevation of extremities, and NSAIDs for pain.
– Lesions heal without ulceration.

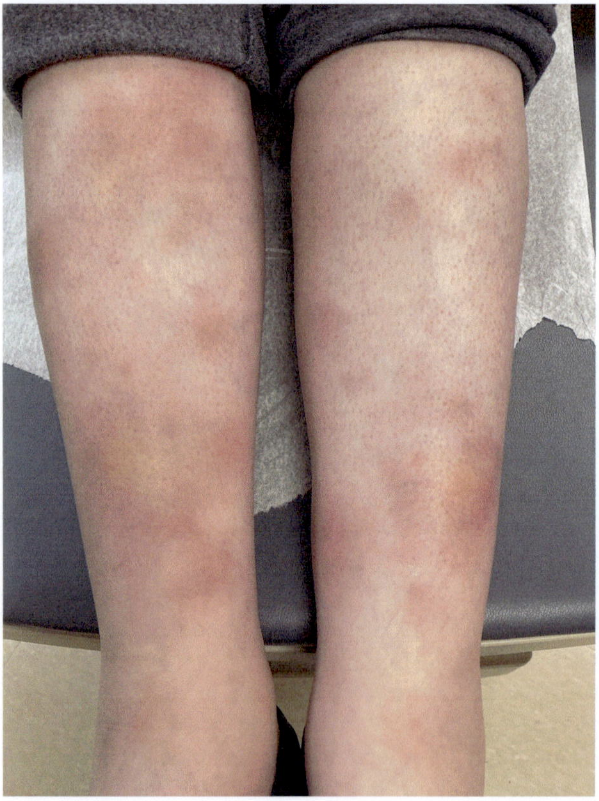

37. Erythrasma

- Morphology/clinical features
  - Thin brown or light pink plaques with fine scale.
  - Fluoresces "coral red" under Wood's lamp.
    - Could be falsely negative if the area was recently washed.
    - In that case, check between the toes with the Wood's lamp.
- Distribution
  - Groin, axilla, inframammary folds, intergluteal, and toe web spaces.
- Etiology/pathogenesis
  - Caused by *Corynebacterium minutissimum* (gram-positive rod).
- Internal sequelae/comorbidities
  - None.
- Laboratory testing
  - None.
- Treatments/prognosis
  - Topical clindamycin or erythromycin
    - Can also use PO erythromycin or tetracyclines in widespread or recalcitrant cases.
- USMLE Board Review Pearls
  - Caused by *Corynebacterium minutissimum* (gram-positive rod).
  - Bacterial coproporphyrin III production is responsible for the "coral red" glow.
  - The wavelength of a Wood's lamp is 365 nm.
    - Note the correct spelling of Wood's lamp.
      - This is named after the physicist Robert W. Wood.

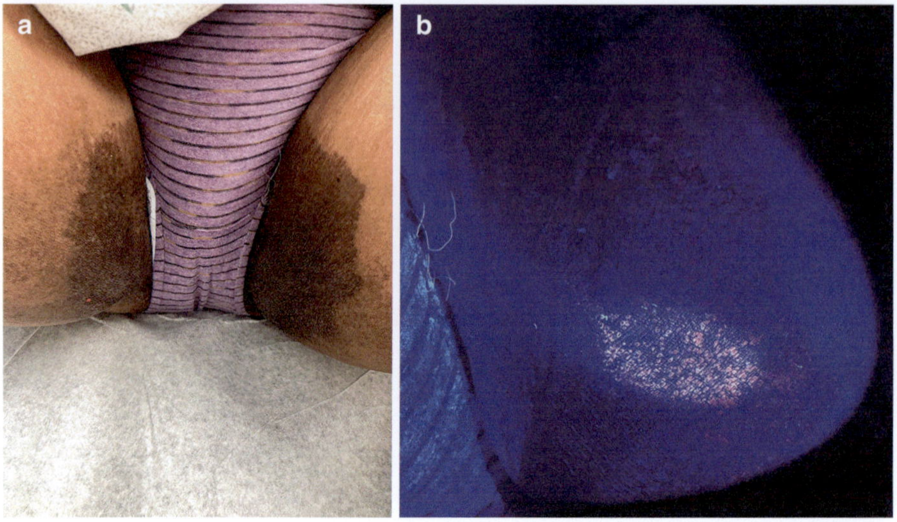

38. Folliculitis

- Morphology/clinical features
  - Follicular-based erythematous pustules.
- Distribution
  - Areas of terminal hair such as scalp, beard, trunk, buttocks, and thighs.
  - Usually multiple.
- Etiology/pathogenesis
  - *Staphylococcus aureus* is the most common cause.
- Internal sequelae/comorbidities
  - None.
- Laboratory testing
  - None.
- Treatments/prognosis
  - PO doxycycline, topical clindamycin, and benzoyl peroxide.
  - Can use Hibiclens skin cleanser wash and mupirocin ointment to the nares for prophylaxis and decolonization of *Staphylococcus aureus*.
- USMLE Board Review Pearls
  - Look for tiny red papules with pinpoint pustules with hair extending from the individual papule.

- Typically caused by infection with *Staphylococcus*, *Streptococcus*, and gram-negative bacteria.
- First-line treatment is topical therapy; for more extensive cases, can use PO antibiotics.
- Hot tub folliculitis is a variant of folliculitis that is caused by *Pseudomonas aeruginosa* from poorly chlorinated whirlpools.
  - Patients will report using a hot tub 1–2 days before the eruption.
  - Look for folliculitis on the trunk (spares shoulders and neck where the patient did not immerse that part of the body).
  - Will resolve on its own.
- Eosinophilic folliculitis is a variant that occurs in AIDS patients.
  - This condition is intensely pruritic.
- Pseudofolliculitis barbae is not a folliculitis in the traditional sense but an inflammatory reaction to tightly coiled hair re-penetrating the skin (usually in African American patients).
  - Commonly referred to as "razor bumps."
  - First step in therapy is to avoid shaving/reduce close shaving.

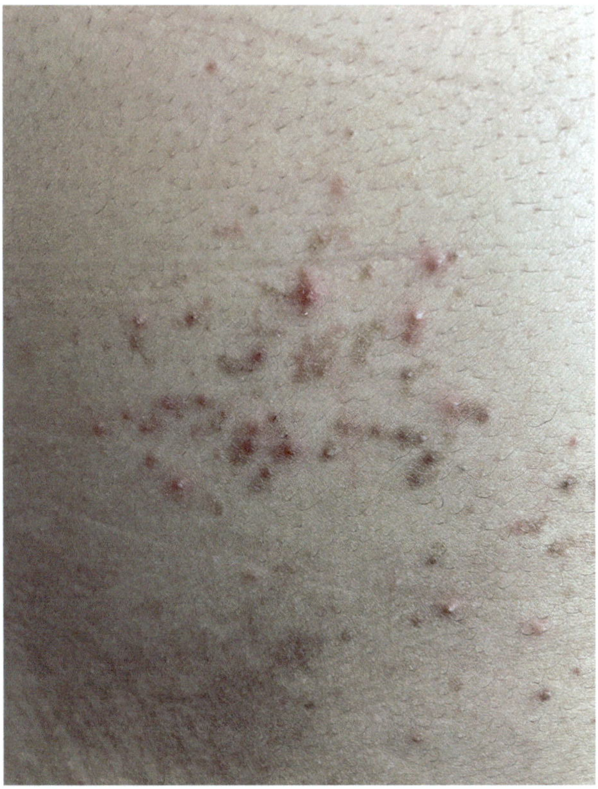

39. Fox–Fordyce disease (apocrine miliaria)

- Morphology/clinical features
  - Skin-colored or yellow-tinged dome-shaped follicular papules.
  - Patients usually complain of pruritus.
- Distribution
  - Most common location is axilla.
    - Can also be seen in periareolar and anogenital regions.
- Etiology/pathogenesis
  - Plugging of apocrine glands.
- Internal sequelae/comorbidities
  - None
- Laboratory testing
  - None.
- Treatments/prognosis
  - Difficult to treat can try tretinoin, topical steroids, topical calcineurin inhibitors, and surgical excision.
  - Can also try OCPs.
- USMLE Board Review Pearls
  - Do not confuse with Fordyce spots, which are ectopic sebaceous glands on the lips/oral mucosa.
  - Look for an adolescent female with numerous skin-colored papules in the axilla; she will complain of pruritus.

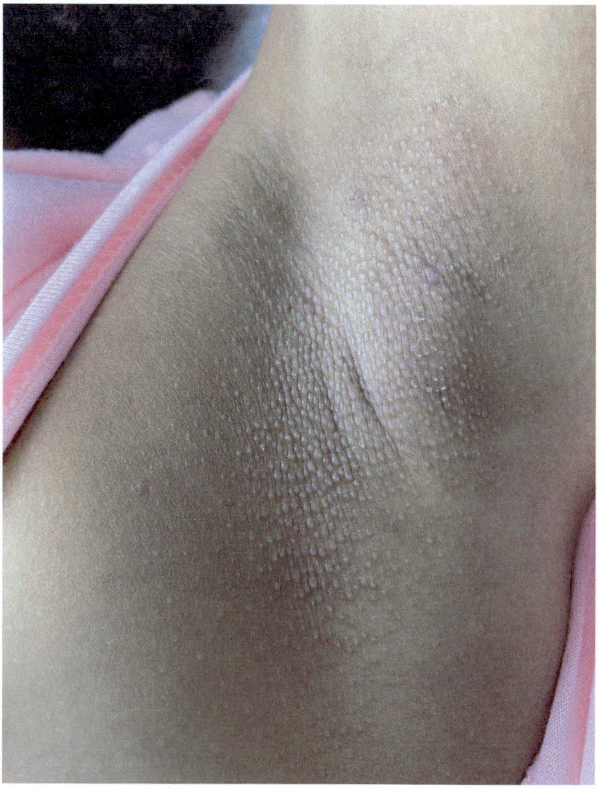

40. Granuloma annulare (GA)

- Morphology/clinical features
  - Annular/arciform nonscaly papules or plaques that range in color from skin-colored to pink to dull red/brown.
  - Patch-type GA lacks an annular configuration and presents as dull red/brown patches and macules on the trunk and extremities.
- Distribution
  - The most common location is on the hands and upper extremity.
    - Specifically seen on the dorsal fingers, hands, and elbows.
  - Can also be seen on the dorsal feet and ankles.
  - Generalized or disseminated presents on the upper trunk and proximal extremities with numerous small dull red/brown nonscaly papules.
- Etiology/pathogenesis
  - Unknown but theorized to occur as a delayed-type hypersensitivity reaction to an unidentified trigger (i.e., trauma, insect bite, infection).

- Internal sequelae/comorbidities
  - No major internal comorbidities.
    - Generalized GA is associated with lipid abnormalities and diabetes.
    - GA-like eruptions have been reported with malignancy.
- Laboratory testing
  - None.
- Treatments/prognosis
  - Spontaneous resolution in 2 years in about 50% of patients with about a 40% risk of recurrence.
  - Difficult to treat but can try topical or intralesional steroids, topical calcineurin inhibitors.
- USMLE Board Review Pearls
  - Look for **nonscaly** papules or plaques on the hands or arms; patients will be asymptomatic.
  - The plaques will likely be in an annular or arciform shape.
  - This condition is difficult to treat effectively; provide reassurance to the patient as to the benign nature of this condition.

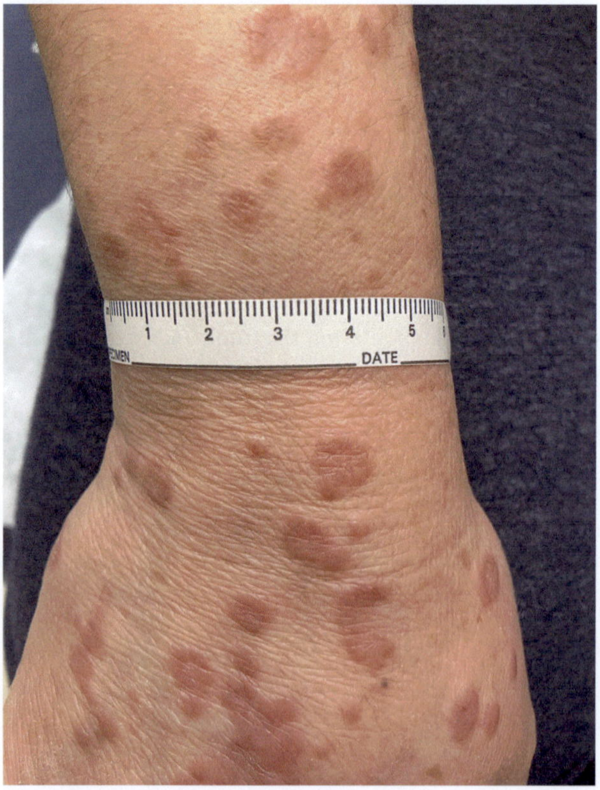

41. Hailey–Hailey disease

- Morphology/clinical features
  - Subtle, flaccid vesicles on normal or inflamed skin that rupture and lead to erythematous macerated/eroded plaques that are malodorous.
  - "Wet tissue paper" appearance.
- Distribution
  - Intertriginous sites commonly involved such as lateral neck, inframammary folds, axillae, groin, and perianal area.
- Etiology/pathogenesis
  - AD mutation in *ATP2C1*
    - Causes defective Ca^{2+} sequestration into Golgi, leading to disturbance in the processing of cell adhesion proteins.
- Internal sequelae/comorbidities
  - Higher risk of secondary infections on the skin.
- Laboratory testing
  - None.
- Treatments/prognosis
  - Difficult to treat!
  - Can try topical steroids and surgical interventions like CO_2 laser.
  - Counsel patient to avoid exacerbating factors like friction, heat, sweat, and adhesive tapes.
- USMLE Board Review Pearls
  - This disease is AD and exhibits complete penetrance and variable expressivity.
  - Age of onset is in the teenage years and early 20s but can arise later in life as well.
  - Mutation: *ATP2C1* (mnemonic: Hailey's Comet—it takes 100 years to see one [2 C 1]).
  - There is no mucosal involvement.
  - Pathology involves the Golgi body at the cellular level.

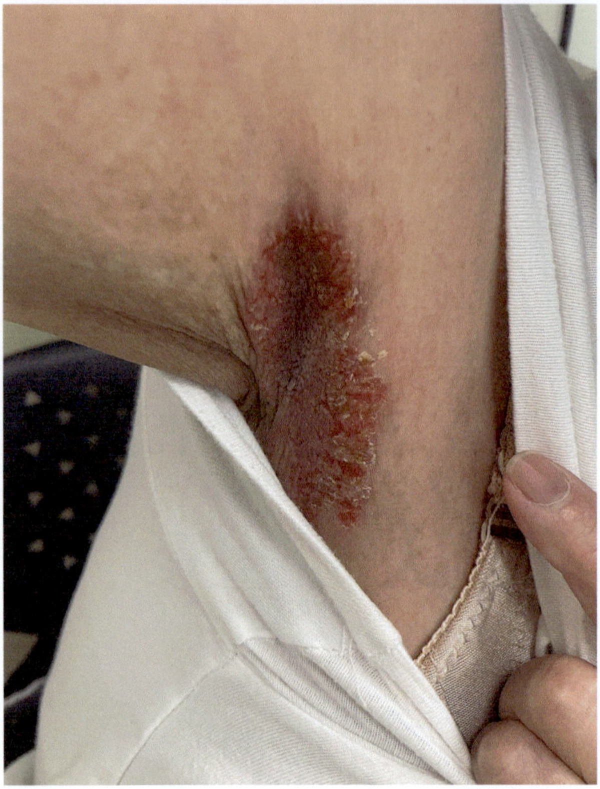

42. Hand-foot-and-mouth disease

- Morphology/clinical features
  - Erythematous macules and oval, deep-seated erythematous vesicles and bullae with gray center.
  - "Football"-shaped vesicles.
  - Patients usually complain of pruritus.
- Distribution
  - Commonly involves palms, soles, buttocks, and oral cavity.
  - More aptly termed "hand, foot, mouth, and butt disease."

- Etiology/pathogenesis
  - Highly infectious!
    - Transmitted by fecal–oral AND respiratory routes.
  - Infection caused by Coxsackie A16 virus (an enterovirus).
    - Coxsackie A6 causes an atypical variant with a more widespread and severe vesiculobullous eruption.
- Internal sequelae/comorbidities
  - a/w onychomadesis (a nail finding) after the infection resolves usually 1–2 months later.
- Laboratory testing
  - None.
- Treatments/prognosis
  - Supportive care.
  - Counsel patients on the infectious nature of condition.
- USMLE Board Review Pearls
  - Look for a viral prodrome (fever, anorexia, oral, and throat pain) and then the characteristic eruption of oral ulcers and a maculopapular/ vesicular rash on the hands and feet and buttocks with "football"-shaped vesicles.
  - Caused by Coxsackie A virus.
    - A nonenveloped single-stranded positive linear RNA virus (picornavirus).
  - Herpangina is a variant of hand, food, and mouth disease, which only involves the oral mucosa (favors the posterior pharynx); patients may have a fever.

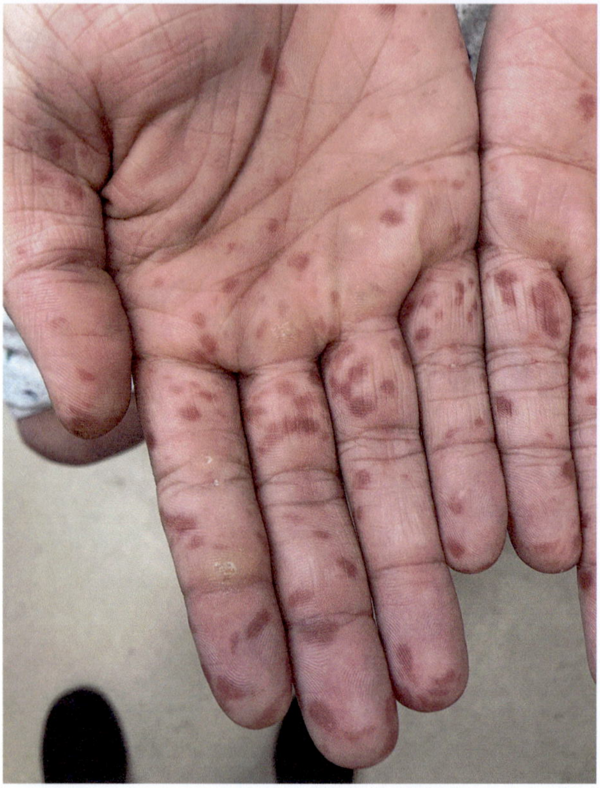

43. Herpes simplex virus

- Morphology/clinical features
  - Grouped vesicles on an erythematous base.
  - Becomes “scalloped ulcers” as the vesicles unroof and heal.
- Distribution
  - Orolabial (classically HSV-1) and anogenital regions (classically HSV-2).
  - Can be seen on the trunk and extremities as well.
  - HSV infection of the fingers is known as herpetic whitlow.
- Etiology/pathogenesis
  - Traditionally HSV-1 is spread by saliva/secretions and HSV-2 is spread by sexual contact. However, there is overlap in that HSV-1 can cause an infection of the anogenital region.
    - Viral replication at skin/mucous membrane leads to retrograde axonal flow to dorsal root ganglia where the virus lays dormant for life and can be reactivated (stress, ultraviolet radiation, fever, injury [i.e., chemical peel or laser surgery], and immunosuppression).

  - Infection can occur without clinical lesions because patients may be shedding virus during the prodrome of a clinical outbreak.
  - It is estimated that approximately one-third of the world's population has experienced a symptomatic HSV infection.
- Internal sequelae/comorbidities
  - Eczema herpeticum is a widespread HSV infection in areas of atopic dermatitis.
  - HSV encephalitis is the most common fatal viral encephalitis in the United States.
  - Can cause congenital and neonatal disease.
  - Ocular HSV.
  - Herpes gladiatorum is an HSV-1 infection from athletic contact.
    - The most common scenario is a wrestler who presents with infection on the lateral neck/face and/or forearm.
- Laboratory testing
  - Viral culture (high Sp, low Sn).
  - PCR of skin lesions (best Sn and Sp).
  - Serologies for antibodies to HSV.
  - Tzanck smear (infrequently used).
    - Bedside test from a vesicle to detect multinucleated giant cells.
- Treatments/prognosis
  - PO valacyclovir for acute flares and prophylaxis of orolabial and anogenital infections.
  - IV acyclovir in severe cases of eczema herpeticum, neonatal HSV, or severe HSV in immunosuppressed patients.
  - Foscarnet or cidofovir for acyclovir-resistant HSV.
- USMLE Board Review Pearls
  - Herpesvirus is an enveloped double-stranded DNA virus.
  - Look for grouped vesicles on an erythematous base around the lips or on the genitals/buttocks. Patients will report burning pain and will report prodromal symptoms of tingling, burning, or pain before an outbreak.
  - HSV-1 classically causes herpes labialis or "cold sores" around the mouth and lips and is triggered by stress, sunlight, or illness.
  - HSV-2 classically causes genital herpes; however, recent data suggests that both HSV-1 and HSV-2 can affect both genital and extragenital (i.e., orolabial) areas.
    - For example, a patient may develop genital herpes if they receive oral sex from a partner who has an active herpes labialis infection (HSV-1) or who is spreading HSV-1 virus in prodromal state without clinical lesions, but this is uncommon and less likely than the traditional way

of contracting a genital herpes infection from a partner with an active genital herpes infection (HSV-2) or one who is spreading HSV-2 virus in a prodromal state without clinical lesions.

- HSV encephalitis most commonly affects the temporal lobe, and HSV-2 is a more common cause of viral meningitis (vs. HSV-1).
- HSV-1 lies dormant most commonly in the trigeminal ganglia, and HSV-2 most commonly lies dormant in the sacral ganglia.
- Outbreaks and suppression can be managed with PO medications but IV acyclovir is the treatment of choice in severe infections, immunosuppressed patients, or infections involving the CNS.
- If a patient is suffering from severe, frequent outbreaks of herpes infection (> 6 outbreaks per year), then daily prophylaxis can be started with PO valacyclovir. In clinical practice, patients are started on prophylaxis more frequently even without the >6 outbreaks per year to reduce viral shedding and recurrences.
  - In addition to decreasing the frequency of symptomatic outbreaks or even eliminating them, suppressive therapy decreases asymptomatic viral shedding by 95% and can thereby reduce transmission of genital herpes to a susceptible partner.
- In HIV/AIDS patients, HSV infections can be persistent and resistant to antiviral therapy.
  - HSV infection lasting greater than 1 month can be considered an AIDS-defining illness.
- Best test is PCR of an unroofed vesicle.

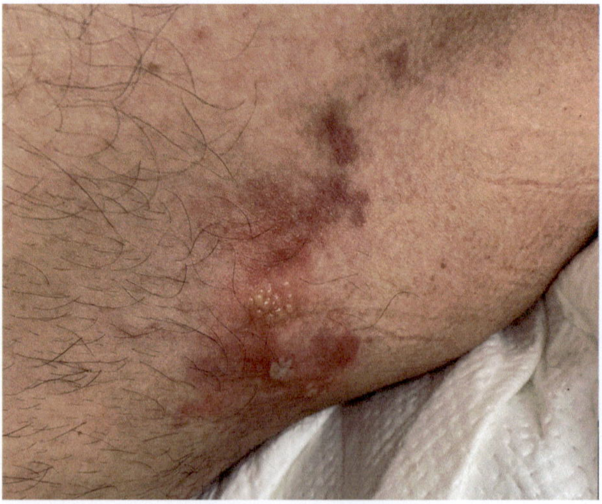

44. Hidradenitis suppurativa

- Morphology/clinical features
  - Recurrent, tender/painful inflammatory nodules, and sterile abscesses a.k.a. "boils" that lead to scarring, sinus tract formation, and doubled-ended comedones.
- Distribution
  - Favors apocrine dense and intertriginous areas.
    - Axilla, inguinal region, intergluteal clefts/buttocks, and inframammary folds.
- Etiology/pathogenesis
  - Combination of follicular occlusion, immune dysregulation, and genetics.
- Internal sequelae/comorbidities
  - A/w obesity, smoking, metabolic syndrome, depression, lymphedema, infections, anemia, and secondary amyloidosis.
- Laboratory testing
  - None.
- Treatments/prognosis
  - Counsel patients to lose weight, stop smoking, and avoid irritating/restricting clothing.
  - PO antibiotics, topical clindamycin, and topical benzoyl peroxide are used to treat flares.
  - Intralesional kenalog, deroofing surgery, and incision & drainage are procedures that can be performed in clinic.
  - FDA-approved biologic therapies are adalimumab (TNF-α inhibitor), secukinumab (IL-17 inhibitor), and bimekizumab (IL-17 inhibitor).
  - Surgery is the only cure.
    - This is a difficult and large procedure performed by a plastic surgeon or general surgeon that requires wide resection of the diseased tissue and skin grafting.
  - Nothing works well for this condition.
- USMLE Board Review Pearls
  - This condition is caused by chronic inflammation of the pilosebaceous unit that leads to inflamed and painful abscesses/nodules with a malodorous discharge that eventually progress to scars and sinus tracts.
  - Look for a patient who complains of waxing/waning and recurring abscesses in the axilla or groin region. They will likely have evidence of

scarring or sinus tract formation on physical exam if they are not currently flaring.
– HS is more common in patients with a family history, African American patients, and patients who are obese or smoke.
– This is a clinical diagnosis, and no lab tests or biopsies are needed.
– First step in management is to counsel patient on weight loss and smoking cessation. Start with oral antibiotics and topical antibiotics (topical clindamycin is first line).

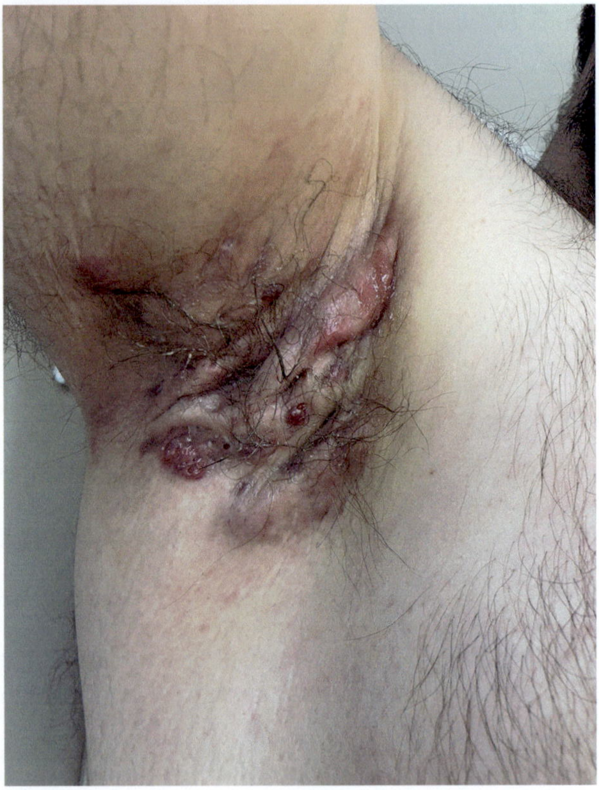

45. Hidrocystoma

- Morphology/clinical features
  - Blue-tinged, translucent cystic papule.
    - Can appear multilocular.
- Distribution
  - Face.
    - Most commonly found in the periocular region.

- Etiology/pathogenesis
  - Apocrine in origin.
- Internal sequelae/comorbidities
  - None.
- Laboratory testing
  - None.
- Treatments/prognosis
  - Surgical excision.
- USMLE Board Review Pearls
  - Look for a bluish, translucent cystic structure near the eye.
  - Will see decapitation secretion on histology.
  - Multiple hidrocystomas are associated with Schöpf–Schulz–Passarge syndrome.
    - This is a genodermatosis a/w multiple hidrocystomas, basal cell carcinomas, syringofibroadenomas, palmoplantar keratoderma, hypodontia, and hypotrichosis.

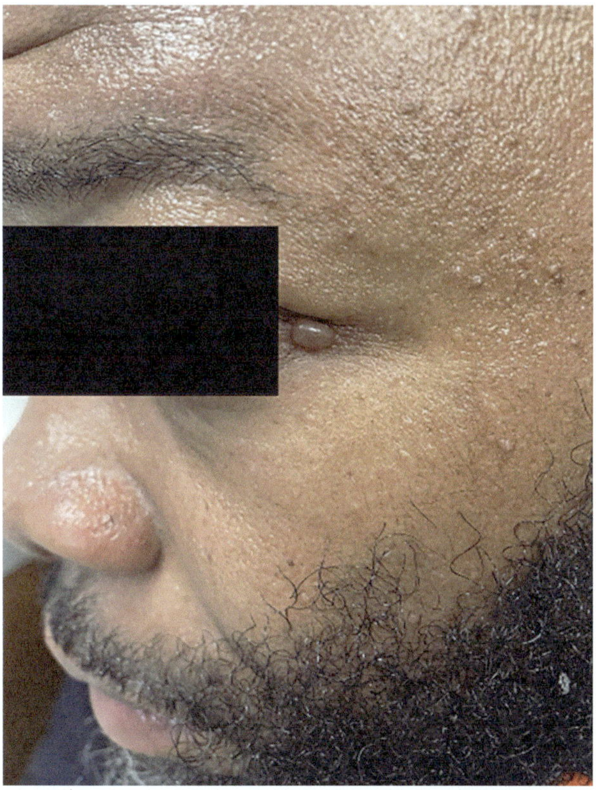

46. Ichthyosis vulgaris

- Morphology/clinical features
  - Fine to large, adherent, dark brown "fish-like" scales.
- Distribution
  - Most commonly seen on the extensor surfaces of lower extremities.
    - The scale on the lower extremities is usually larger.
    - Can also be seen on the trunk.
- Etiology/pathogenesis
  - A disorder of cornification due to a filaggrin mutation.
- Internal sequelae/comorbidities
  - A/w atopic dermatitis, keratosis pilaris, and hyperlinear palms.
- Laboratory testing
  - This is a clinical diagnosis but can perform genetic testing for *FLG* mutation.
- Treatments/prognosis
  - Use of emollients, humectants, and keratolytic agents to reduce scaling.
    - These agents include topical urea and/or glycolic, lactic, or salicylic acid.
    - There is no effective treatment or cure.
- USMLE Board Review Pearls
  - Look for dark brown, medium to large, well-defined, "fish-like" adherent scales on the extensor extremities of the lower extremities.
    - Ichthyosis is Greek for "fish-like."
  - Due to a mutation in the filaggrin gene (*FLG*).
  - Clinical diagnosis, treat with emollients and moisturizers.
  - Begins in infancy or early childhood.
  - Associated with atopic dermatitis.

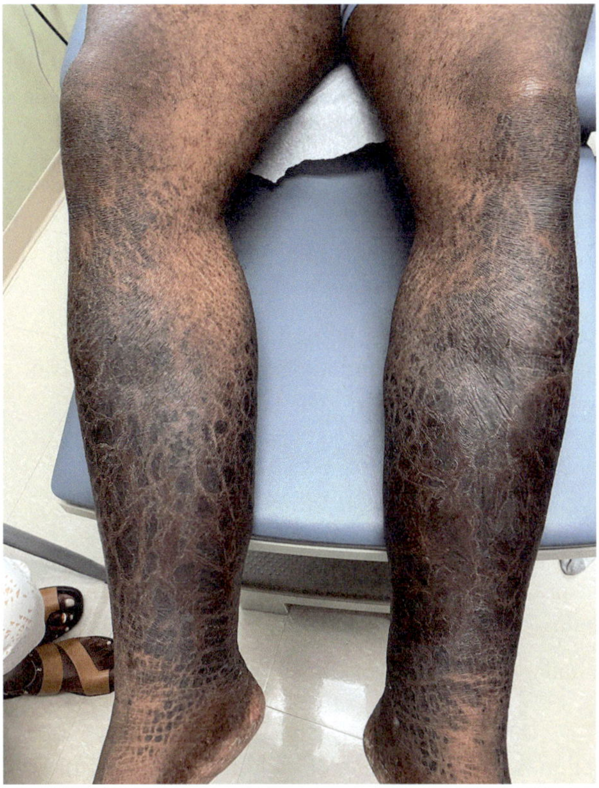

47. Impetigo

- Morphology/clinical features/distribution
  - Nonbullous impetigo—erosions, pustules, and honey-colored crusts most commonly seen around the perinasal and perioral areas.
  - Bullous impetigo—flaccid round bullae and erosions with collarettes of scale with minimal surrounding erythema, can be seen on the trunk and extremities.
  - Ecthyma—deeper variant of impetigo that presents with a vesicopustule that develops into a punched-out ulcer with a hemorrhagic/necrotic base most commonly seen on the legs.
- Etiology/pathogenesis
  - *Staph* and *strep* bacteria
    - Impetigo is more commonly caused by *staph.*

    - Ecthyma is more commonly caused by *strep*.
  - Bullous impetigo is caused by *S. aureus* phage group II (types 55 and 71), which produces exfoliatoxins A and B, leading to cleavage of desmoglein 1 that results in a blister.
- Internal sequelae/comorbidities
  - In 5% of cases, nonbullous impetigo caused by *strep* (M protein types 1, 4, 12, 49, 55, 57, 60) results in acute poststreptococcal glomerulonephritis (APSG).
    - Risk is not altered by antibiotic therapy.
    - No known risk of rheumatic fever from this infection.
- Laboratory testing
  - None.
- Treatments/prognosis
  - Localized—topical mupirocin, retapamulin.
  - Widespread—oral β-lactamase resistant penicillin or first-generation cephalosporin.
    - Clindamycin or doxycycline if patient fails therapy.
- USMLE Board Review Pearls
  - Impetigo is a superficial infection of the epidermis that is caused by both *staph* and *strep* bacteria; it is common in children and spreads by direct contact and could spread quickly in an infected patient—very contagious!
  - Look for erythematous plaques with "honey-colored" crusts around the nose or mouth in a pediatric patient.
  - This is a clinical diagnosis, could perform a gram stain or culture to identify causative organism, but this is not necessary to begin therapy.
  - Treat mild disease with topical therapy (mupirocin) and treat severe and widespread disease with oral antibiotics (cephalexin or dicloxacillin).
  - The patient may return to school 24 hours after initiation of therapy as long as they are feeling well and the affected areas are covered.
  - Complications include acute poststreptococcal glomerulonephritis (APSG).

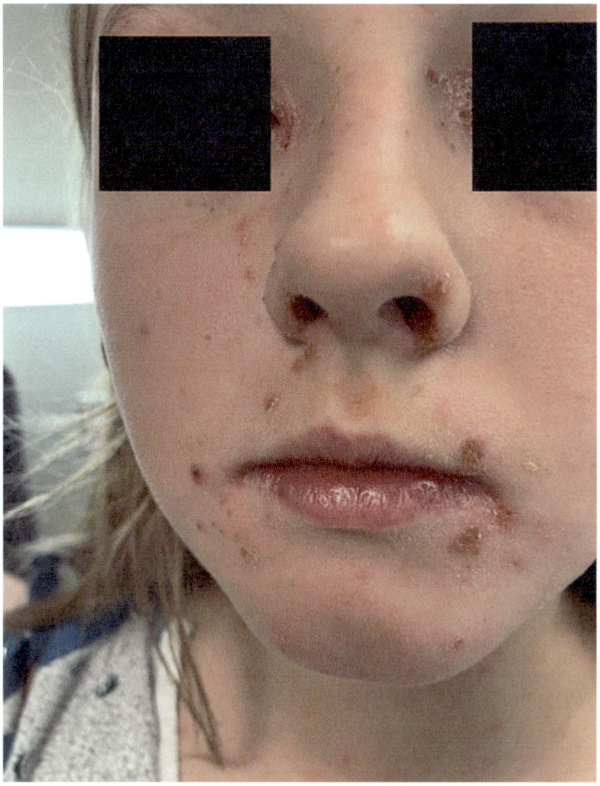

48. Infantile hemangioma

- Morphology/clinical features
  - Bright red "vascular appearing" lobulated papule.
  - Deeper hemangiomas have a purple/blue color with no overlying skin change.
- Distribution
  - Anywhere (including mucosal surfaces).
    - Most commonly seen on the trunk and head/neck region.
- Etiology/pathogenesis
  - Abnormal vascular development and proliferation.

    - Stems from de novo formation of vessels from multipotent hemangioma-derived stem cells (HemSCs), endothelial progenitor cells, as well as the formation of new vessels from existing ones.

- Internal sequelae/comorbidities
  - Hemangiomas in a "beard distribution" may involve the airway.
  - Periorbital hemangiomas may cause astigmatism or amblyopia.
  - Liver is the most common site of internal hemangiomas, and ultrasound is recommended when ≥5 skin lesions are present. Liver involvement could rarely lead to consumptive hypothyroidism.
- Laboratory testing
  - None.
- Treatments/prognosis
  - In many cases, a "watch and wait approach" is reasonable for small, uncomplicated hemangiomas (ensure there is no cosmetic or functional concern) as standard teaching is that 50% involute by 5 years of age and 90% by 9 years of age.
  - Can treat with topical timolol or oral propranolol for lesions that may lead to poor cosmetic outcomes or are impacting function.
- USMLE Board Review Pearls
  - Infantile hemangiomas are GLUT-1 positive and are not fully formed at birth as opposed to RICH and NICH (GLUT-1 negative and are fully formed at birth).
    - RICH = rapidly involuting congenital hemangioma.
    - NICH = noninvoluting congenital hemangioma.
  - Infantile hemangiomas can spontaneously involute, cherry angiomas do not have this ability.
  - Involution typically begins at 9 months to 1 year of age.
  - Perform liver ultrasound if a patient has ≥5 skin lesions.

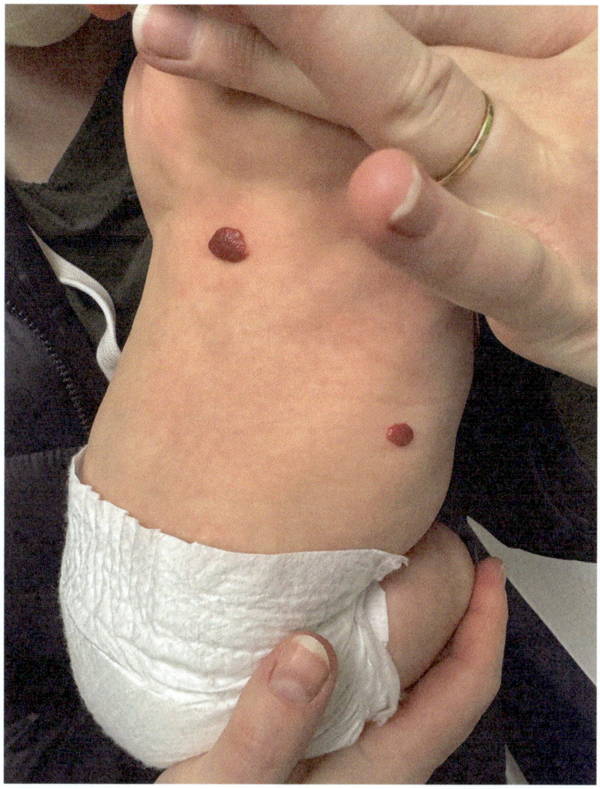

49. Infundibular cyst

- Morphology/clinical features
  - Skin-colored nodule with central punctum.
    - Sometimes the punctum is not obvious.
  - Also called epidermoid cyst or epidermal inclusion cyst.
- Distribution
  - Can be seen anywhere but most commonly seen on the head, neck, and trunk.
- Etiology/pathogenesis
  - Cyst that is derived from the infundibulum of the hair follicle.
- Internal sequelae/comorbidities
  - None.

- Multiple infundibular cysts may be a/w Gardner syndrome; these cysts classically have pilomatricoma-like changes histologically.

- Laboratory testing
  - None.
- Treatments/prognosis
  - Surgical excision with removal of the capsule.
- USMLE Board Review Pearls
  - Look for a firm or freely mobile cyst surrounding a hair follicle with a central punctum.
    - May become infected characterized by acute erythema, pain/tenderness, and drainage
      - Treat with incision and drainage and PO antibiotics.
  - Does not dimple when pinched (as opposed to a dermatofibroma).
  - Patients may report a "cheese-like," odoriferous discharge.

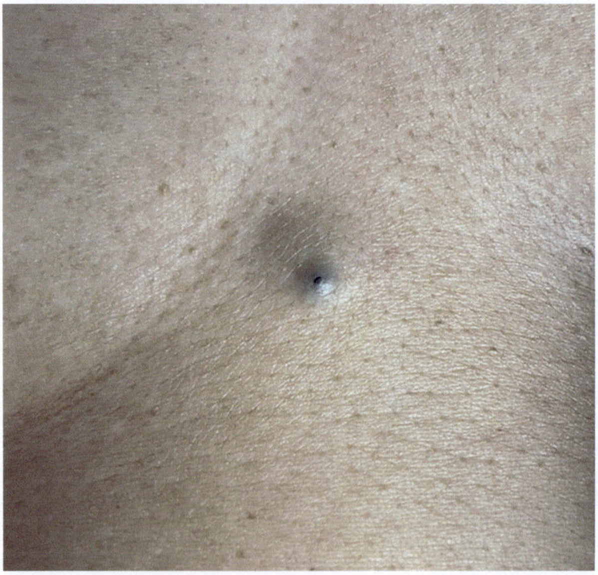

50. Kaposi sarcoma (KS)

- Morphology/clinical features
  - Violaceous plaque, patch, or nodule.

- Distribution
  - Classic KS initially starts on the distal extremities in elderly men of Mediterranean or Ashkenazi Jewish descent.
  - AIDS-associated KS is located on the trunk and midface.
- Etiology/pathogenesis
  - NOT A SARCOMA (malignancy) in the traditional sense of the word, although it can behave aggressively requiring chemotherapy.
  - This is an HHV-8-driven vascular proliferation with variable clinical relevance.
- Internal sequelae/comorbidities
  - Can progress systemically to involve visceral organs or involve the lymph nodes.
- Laboratory testing
  - Nuclear positivity (on immunohistochemistry) for latency-associated nuclear antigen (LANA-1) of HHV-8 is extremely helpful diagnostically (nearly 100% sensitive and specific).
- Treatments/prognosis
  - Difficult to treat effectively.
    - Can try cryosurgery, laser surgery, topical alitretinoin gel, and radiation therapy.
    - KS does not require treatment if localized on the skin with no impact on function.
    - Systemic chemotherapy is needed for rapidly progressing systemic KS.
- USMLE Board Review Pearls
  - Classically seen in older Eastern European males, patients with AIDS, and organ transplant patients.
    - Looks for the characteristic morphology within these patient populations.
  - A vascular proliferative disease caused by HHV-8.
  - Systemic involvement can be seen in the GI tract and lungs.
  - The incidence of HIV-associated KS has decreased in the age of HAART therapy.
    - If the patient is HIV positive, the initial preferred therapy is initiation of HAART therapy.
  - Systemic chemotherapy of choice for aggressive or internal disease is doxorubicin, paclitaxel, or interferon-α.

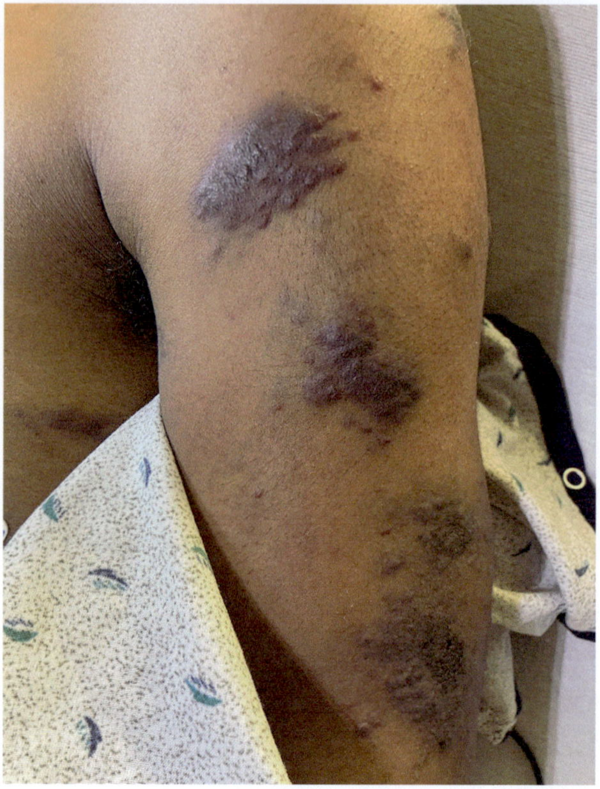

51. Keloid

- Morphology/clinical features
  - Firm, raised, smooth, hairless, and shiny papules or plaques that are ovoid, round, or geometric in shape.
  - Usually not confined to wound margins and can grow outside of the original injury.
- Distribution
  - Most commonly seen on the neck, ears, extremities, lower abdomen, shoulder, and upper chest (especially the pre-sternal area).
- Etiology/pathogenesis
  - Aberrant wound healing and excessive scar formation mainly due to increased TGF-β level signaling.

- Internal sequelae/comorbidities
  - None.
- Laboratory testing
  - None.
- Treatments/prognosis
  - There is a high rate of recurrence with excision alone.
    - Must perform either intralesional steroid, radiation therapy, or intralesional imiquimod after excision to help prevent/mitigate recurrence.
  - Intralesional steroids are used to help shrink and flatten the keloid and treat the pruritus associated with the keloid.
- USMLE Board Review Pearls
  - Increased TGF-β levels are a/w keloid formation.
  - On exams, the questions will usually test your knowledge of a keloid vs. a hypertrophic scar.
    - Keloids extend beyond the original wound and are commonly seen on the earlobes, face, chest, and upper extremities while a hypertrophic scar is red and raised but confined to the original wound or incision.
    - Recurrence is infrequent after removal of a hypertrophic scar but keloids frequently recur after excision without additional intervention.
    - Keloids are more frequent in African American patients. Keloids can spontaneously form without history of injury while a hypertrophic scar cannot and must precede injury.
    - A hypertrophic scar is classically very erythematous while a keloid may not be. Hypertrophic scars usually form within weeks to months of injury while keloids may have a more delayed onset.
  - Scars never regain full tensile strength. The maximum tensile strength a scar will obtain is 80% of baseline.

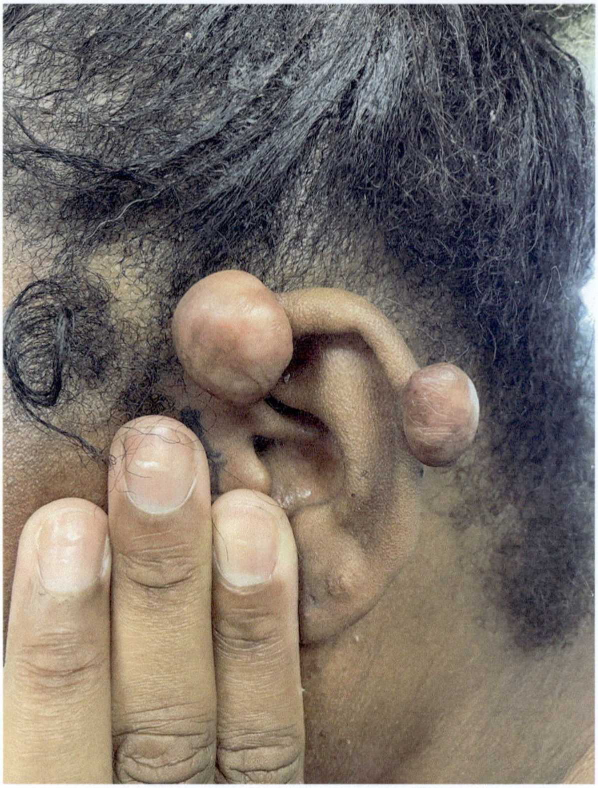

52. Leprosy

- Morphology/clinical features
  - There is a wide variety of clinical findings in leprosy!
    - You should suspect leprosy when a patient is from another country or has extensive travel history with various dermatological findings that "you can't put together."
  - Classic and nearly pathognomonic findings include anesthesia in a hypopigmented or erythematous skin lesion and enlarged peripheral nerves with associated loss of sensation or weakness.
  - Late findings in lepromatous leprosy (LL) are characterized by madarosis (loss of eyelashes or eyebrows), saddle nose, infiltration of the earlobes, acquired ichthyosis of lower extremities, and lagophthalmos.
    - These findings are collectively referred to as "leonine facies" (the patient's face looks like a lion).

  - Tuberculoid leprosy classically presents with a few patches or plaques that have sharply demarcated, slightly raised borders and lesional alopecia and anesthesia are often present.
- Distribution
  - Commonly involves the face, trunk, and extremities.
- Etiology/pathogenesis
  - Mycobacterial infection from *M. leprae* and *M. lepromatosis*
    - Small, obligate intracellular slightly curved bacterial rods that are acid fast.
- Internal sequelae/comorbidities
  - Neuropathic changes (sensory and motor), vasomotor alterations, and secretory disturbances (dry skin and eyes).
- Laboratory testing
  - Skin biopsy demonstrating bacilli.
  - PCR.
  - Cannot be cultured in vitro by traditional methods.
- Treatments/prognosis
  - Multidrug therapy is extremely effective.
  - The WHO 2018 guidelines recommend a three-drug regimen consisting of rifampin, dapsone, and clofazimine for all patients with leprosy, with a treatment duration of 6 months for paucibacillary (PB) disease and 12 months for multibacillary (MB) disease.
  - Patients may be referred to Hansen's Disease Ambulatory Care Clinics (https://www.hrsa.gov/hansens-disease/ambulatory-clinics) for referral to one of 900 private physicians nationwide who have expertise in treating leprosy.
    - Phone 1-800-642-2477, weekdays 9 a.m. to 5:30 p.m. ET.
- USMLE Board Review Pearls
  - Look for a patient from another country, a patient with extensive travel history, or a patient who has had contact with an armadillo (usually a veterinarian or a zoo-worker).
    - The highest incidence is seen in the following countries: Brazil, India, Nepal, Indonesia, and Bangladesh.
  - Leprosy is also called Hansen's disease, and it is caused by *M. leprae,* which is an acid-fast bacillus that has a predilection for cooler temperature (this is why peripheral nerves are impacted in a "glove and stocking" distribution and structures such as nose and ears are impacted).

- The reservoir in the United States for this bacterium is the armadillo.
- There are two forms of leprosy to be aware of:
  - On the exam, lepromatous leprosy will likely present diffusely with leonine facies. These patients have a very high bacterial load, are contagious, and have a low cell-mediated immunity that is characterized by a response from the Th_2 immune arm.
    - Lepromatous leprosy has **2** Ls and is characterized by $\mathbf{Th_2}$ immune response.
    - **L**epromatous leprosy is more **L**ethal.
      - Higher bacterial load and more skin involvement.
  - On the exam, tuberculoid leprosy will present with one or a few anesthetic or alopecic hypopigmented or erythematous skin plaques. These patients have a high cell-mediated immunity, low bacterial load, and an immune response that is characterized by a response from the Th_1 immune arm.

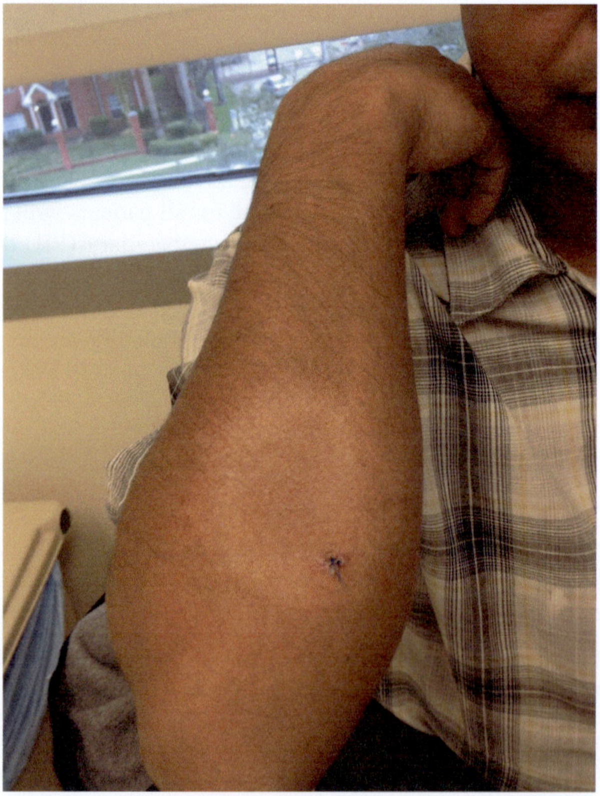

53. Leukocytoclastic vasculitis

- Morphology/clinical features
  - Crops/groups of numerous partially blanchable, symmetric "palpable purpura."
    - The areas appear bruised-like but can be palpated (sometimes this can be very subtle or almost nonexistent).
  - Rare manifestations include vesicles, pustules, bullae, round ulcers, targetoid lesions, and erythematous papules/plaques.
- Distribution
  - Most commonly seen on lower extremities.
  - Can also be seen on the trunk and upper extremities in dependent areas or areas under occlusion (i.e., tight clothing).
- Etiology/pathogenesis
  - This is a small vessel vasculitis.
    - Caused by immune complex deposition in post-capillary venules that leads to inflammation and vessel damage.
  - Most cases (nearly 50%) are idiopathic.
    - Other causes include infections, systemic inflammatory/autoimmune diseases, medications, and malignancies.
      - Common examples to be aware of include *strep* infection, hepatitis, antibiotics, NSAIDs, hematologic malignancies, and autoimmune connective tissue diseases (SLE, Sjögren's disease, rheumatoid arthritis).
- Internal sequelae/comorbidities
  - None.
    - Can be associated with systemic inflammatory/autoimmune diseases or malignancies.
- Laboratory testing
  - In the appropriate context, patients may need an extensive workup with physical exam and laboratory testing. Can consider CBC, BMP, ESR, LFTs, UA, stool guaiac, ANA, RF, complement levels, SPEP/UPEP, Hep B/C, HIV, ASO titer, CXR, and cultures based on history.
- Treatments/prognosis
  - Good prognosis, 10% may have a chronic or relapsing/remitting course.
  - If severe symptoms or a protracted course, can give PO steroid taper over 4–6 weeks.

- USMLE Board Review Pearls
  - Look for palpable purpura on the lower extremities with an acute onset.
  - Commonly occurs 7–10 days after an implicated medication.
    - Look for penicillin, cephalosporins, and sulfonamides in the question stem or answer choices.
    - Also look for infections, including HCV and HIV, in the question stem or answer choices.

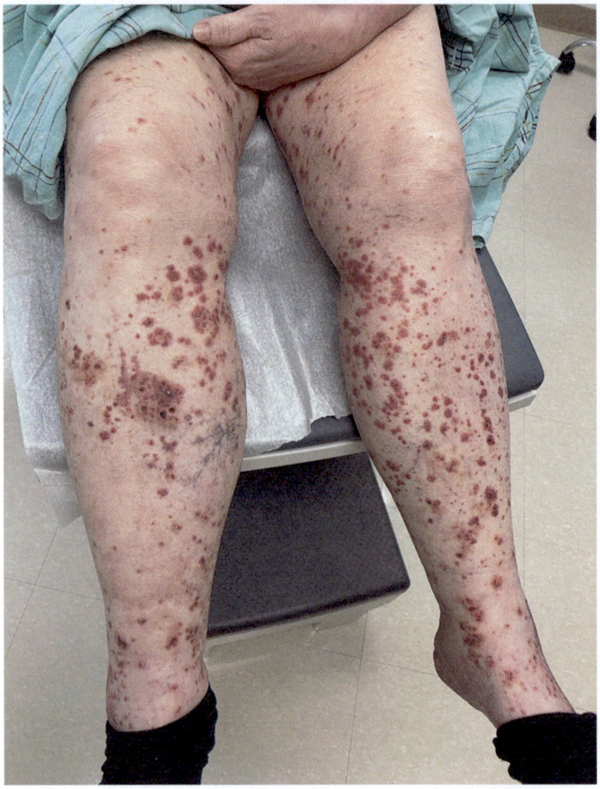

54. Lice

- Morphology/clinical features/distribution
  - Head lice—patients with head lice present with pruritus concentrated to the scalp, behind the ears and nape of the neck. Nits (egg capsules) can be seen as small (0.8mm), firm, adherent nodules on the hair shaft.
  - Body lice—patients with body lice present with severe pruritus and often have pinpoint red macules, small erythematous papules, crusts, and excoriations. Nits and adult lice are often found on the patients' clothing seams.

- Public lice—also known as crabs or crab lice usually presents as pruritus in the pubic region and can be brown to skin-colored and mimic hemorrhagic crusts. Erythema around the follicles can be seen.
- Macula caerulea are asymptomatic, slate-gray to bluish irregular-shaped macules that measure 0.5–1cm on the trunk and thighs.
  - Theorized to result from breakdown of bilirubin to biliverdin by enzymes in louse saliva.

- Etiology/pathogenesis
  - Lice are bloodsucking, wingless insects.
  - Head lice = *Pediculus capitis*, crab lice = *Pthirus pubis,* body lice = *Pediculus humanus var. corporis.*
- Internal sequelae/comorbidities
  - None.
- Laboratory testing
  - None.
  - Lice and nits can be seen with the naked eye on the body and clothing.
- Treatments/prognosis
  - Crab lice = PO ivermectin, topical permethrin, lindane shampoo.
  - Head lice = PO ivermectin, topical spinosad, topical permethrin, malathion lotion, or gel.
    - Usually, the nits need to be removed with a specialized nit comb.
    - A clinical trial (n = 1038) showed that 0.9% spinosad suspension left on for 10 minutes without nit combing on day 1 +/- day 7 had superior efficacy to 1% permethrin cream with nit combing.
  - Body lice = MUST TREAT/WASH/CHANGE CLOTHES OR BEDDING, the patient will not get better if the source is not eradicated as body lice live on the clothes or bedding [must wash in hot water ≥130°F and dry in hot heat dryer].
- USMLE Board Review Pearls
  - Look for a patient with pruritus behind the ears or in the pubic region. A patient with body lice will usually be homeless (they cannot wash their clothes or bedding). Lice are visible to the naked eye but a dermatoscope helps in identification.
  - Lice are commonly spread through body contact, sharing of clothes/bedding, sharing of hair accessories, or combs/brushes.
  - Classroom breakouts of head lice can be seen (head lice is also known as "cooties").

- Body lice are the vector for the following infectious diseases: *Rickettsia prowazekii* (epidemic typhus), *Borrelia recurrentis* (relapsing fever), and *Bartonella quintana* (trench fever).
- Crab lice can affect the eyelashes; if a pediatric patient presents with these findings, then suspicion should be raised for sexual abuse.
- Treatment of choice for body lice is to treat the clothes and bedding and not primarily treat the patient with medications (rarely topical permethrin is needed for the patient).
- The incidence of crab lice has decreased with current cultural practices of hair removal from the pubic/genital region.

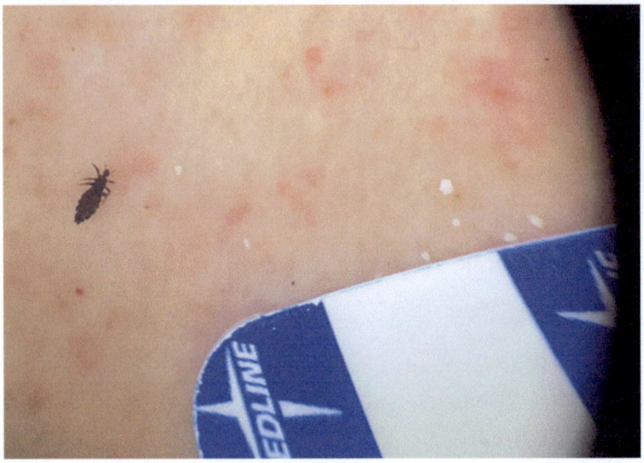

55. Lichen planus

- Morphology/clinical features
  - 5 Ps—"pruritic, planar (flat-topped), purple/violaceous, polygonal, papules."
    - While the color is classically a purple/violaceous one, they are sometimes a dull red color.
  - Papules may be umbilicated.
  - Characteristically exhibit Wickham's striae, which is a slightly shiny and transparent network of fine white lines.
  - Koebnerization seen often.
  - There are numerous clinical variants of LP that include annular, erosive, atrophic, drug-induced, hypertrophic, linear, nail, inverse, lichen planopilaris, and LP pigmentosus.
- Distribution
  - Classicly affects ventral wrists/forearms, dorsal hands, genitalia, and presacral area.

  - Oral mucosae commonly involved.
    - Look for Wickham's striae on buccal mucosal or lips.
- Etiology/pathogenesis
  - T-cell-mediated autoimmune damage to keratinocytes that express altered self-antigens on their surface from a variety of triggers, including viral, contact allergens, medications, or idiopathic.
    - To put it another way, there is a cross-reaction/molecular mimicry of T-cells to exogenous antigens in the epidermis that are usually not recognized by T-cells.
  - Hepatitis C virus has been specifically implicated.
  - Drug-induced LP = HCTZ, β-blockers, ACEi, antimalarials.
- Internal sequelae/comorbidities
  - There is an increased risk of SCC progression in hypertrophic LP, oral ulcerative LP, and vulvovaginal LP.
- Laboratory testing
  - None.
- Treatments/prognosis
  - Many forms will resolve on their own (1–2 years).
    - Exception is oral, hypertrophic, or nail.
  - Treatments include topical corticosteroids, methotrexate, acitretin, oral metronidazole, but there are no highly effective therapies.
- USMLE Board Review Pearls
  - Look for purple/violaceous flat-topped papules/plaques in a polygonal (many straight sides) shape on the wrists or presacral area. Patients will likely complain of pruritus.
  - Also look for lacy white lines (Wickham's striae) and Koebner phenomena.
    - Koebner will likely appear as LP developing in or following an area where the patient scratched their skin.
  - LP is associated with hepatitis C infection, and common drug triggers on exams include thiazides, quinines, and β-blockers.
  - Treat mild and limited disease with topical corticosteroids and severe/generalized disease with systemic therapy.
  - The dermatopathology is highly testable = sawtooth (sharp or point-like areas of epidermis) rete ridges with lichenoid infiltrate (lymphocytes infiltrating the dermo-epidermal junction obscuring the normal sharply demarcated border). In some areas of the epidermis, there will be

hypergranulosis (the granular layer will appear deep purple, more prominent, and expanded).

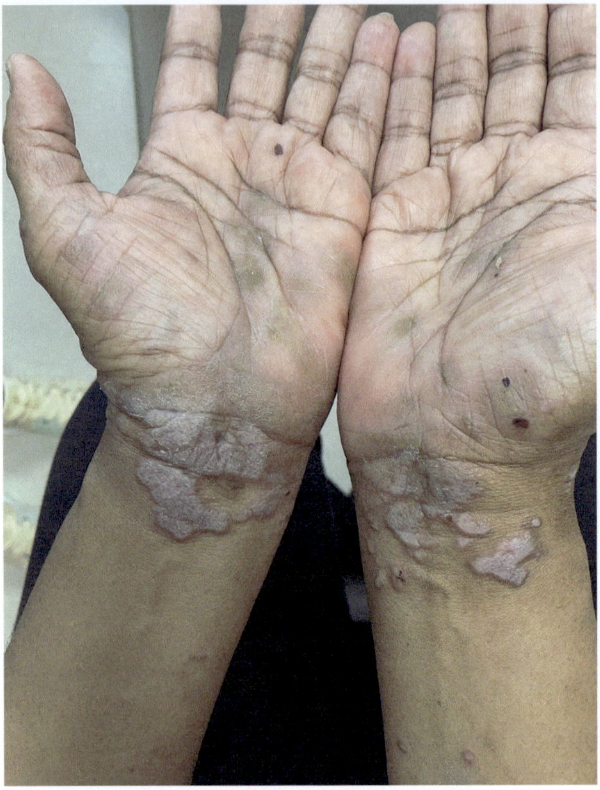

56. Mastocytosis (cutaneous)

- Morphology/clinical features/distribution
  - Solitary mastocytoma—single red/yellowish/brown plaque or nodule usually on the extremities.
  - Maculopapular cutaneous mastocytosis—multiple light brown/red brown macules and papules on the trunk and extremities (spares palms, face, and soles).
    - Most common presentation in children.
  - Diffuse cutaneous mastocytosis—large edematous, peau d'orange plaques involving large areas of the skin that frequently blister leading to erosions.
  - Adult form is characterized by reddish-brown papules and macules on the trunk and extremities.
  - Telangiectasia macularis eruptive perstans (TMEP) is a rare variant characterized by patches of telangiectasias with no hyperpigmentation.
    - TMEP is overdiagnosed; it is rare.

  - Darier's sign = local erythema or an urticarial wheal forming after friction or rubbing. This is a characteristic physical exam finding. Do not confuse with Darier disease.
- Etiology/pathogenesis
  - Alterations in KIT structure and activity are central to the pathogenesis of mastocytosis.
- Internal sequelae/comorbidities
  - In children, there are rarely internal manifestations.
  - In adults, systemic manifestations include bone marrow involvement, hepatosplenomegaly, GI symptoms, and even mixed organic brain syndrome (constellation of symptoms, including irritability, fatigue, headache, poor attention span).
- Laboratory testing
  - Serum α and β tryptase levels.
- Treatments/prognosis
  - For pediatric macrocytosis, the prognosis is good; the treatment mainly consists of counseling and the avoidance of certain provocative factors.
    - Patients should avoid the following triggers. The triggers can be remembered with the mnemonic "PROMS" (**P**olymyxin, **R**adiocontrast dye/**R**um [alcohol], **O**pioids, **M**uscle relaxants, **S**alicylates/nSaid**S**).
    - Acetaminophen is safe to take for a mastocytosis patient.
  - The treatment and prognosis of adult mastocytosis depends on the extent of systemic involvement and are beyond the scope of this book.
- USMLE Board Review Pearls
  - This is an uncommon and interesting disorder defined as an excess of mast cells in the skin or other systemic organs.
  - Look for few to numerous red/brown maculopapular lesions.
  - Mast cells are responsible for allergic reactions in tissues and can bind the Fc portion of IgE to their cell membrane (FcεRI). When a specific antigen binds to mast cell-bound IgE, the FcεRI becomes activated. This leads to degranulation and release of preformed mediators (such as histamine and serotonin) leading to a characteristic physiologic response.
  - Degranulation causes release of histamine, heparin, and tryptase. Some mediators are preformed and others are not (they are newly synthesized i.e. prostaglandins and leukotrienes).
  - Mastocytosis is a/w a *c-KIT* mutation.
  - Common signs/symptoms in adults with systemic involvement include flushing, pruritus, hypotension, abdominal pain, and diarrhea.
    - Systemic involvement is rare in children.

- Treatment involves counseling on prevocational factors but medications that prevent mast cell degranulation may be used, including cromolyn, antileukotrienes, and antihistamines.
- Darier's sign = formation of local erythema or urticarial wheal, after friction or rubbing, is characteristic.
- Mast cells stain with the following: toluidine blue, Giemsa, Leder, tryptase, and CD117 (kit) antibodies.

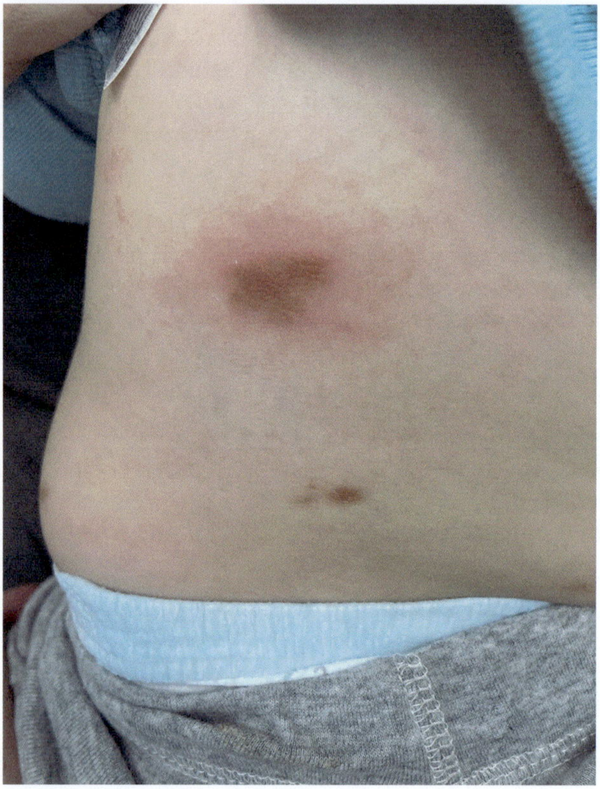

57. Melanoma

- Morphology/clinical features/distribution
  - Melanoma can have many different morphologies or clinical features. Classically the ABCDE (**A**symmetry, **B**order irregular, **C**olor variations, **D**iameter > 6 mm, **E**volution or change in the lesion) mnemonic has been used to identify concerning lesions for both clinicians and patients. Many of these criteria apply to noncancerous lesions such as a seborrheic keratosis or a dysplastic nevus. The following general "rules of thumb" will help guide the clinician on what requires a biopsy. These rules

do not supersede the experience of a well-trained, board-certified dermatologist.

- If it stands out, then biopsy it (also known as the "ugly duckling sign").
- If the lesion is new, rapidly changing, growing, or bleeding.
- If the patient points out a lesion to you and it's not stone-cold normal, then it should probably be sampled.
- There should be a lower threshold to biopsy anything on an older patient with a history of significant sun damage.

– Be aware of amelanotic melanoma (lacking clinically evident pigment), desmoplastic melanoma (skin-colored/pink/red nodule on sun-exposed skin), and acral lentiginous melanoma (ALM, represents a disproportionate percentage of melanomas diagnosed in Black, Asian [up to 22%], and Hispanic patients).
– The 2023 WHO Classification of Skin Tumors now recognizes nine major subtypes of melanoma based on their proposed pathogenesis: (1) low-chronic sun-damaged skin (CSD) melanoma; (2) lentigo maligna melanoma (high-CSD melanoma); (3) desmoplastic melanoma; (4) Spitz melanoma; (5) acral melanoma; (6) mucosal melanoma; (7) melanoma arising in a giant congenital nevus; (8) melanoma arising in a blue nevus; and (9) ocular (uveal, conjunctival) melanoma.
– Superficial spreading melanoma is commonly seen on the trunk and legs, nodular melanoma is most commonly seen on head/neck, lentigo maligna is most commonly seen on CSD skin of head and neck.
– ALM is most commonly seen in darkly pigmented races and characteristically displays Hutchinson's sign, which is hyperpigmentation extending onto the hyponychium or beyond the lateral or proximal nail fold.

- Etiology/pathogenesis
  – Risk factors include lightly pigmented skin, UV exposure (both short intermittent, intense exposure, and cumulative exposure), large number of acquired and dysplastic melanocytic nevi, solar lentigines, freckles, and red hair.
  – Familial atypical mole and melanoma syndrome, also known as FAMM syndrome (inherited *CDKN2A* mutation).
  – Genetic mutations such as BRAF V600E in superficial spreading melanoma.
- Internal sequelae/comorbidities
  – Risk of metastasis to internal organs.
- Laboratory testing
  – Need to biopsy the lesion to determine the Breslow thickness, which is one of the most important factors in tumor staging.

- Treatments/prognosis
  - Prognosis highly depends on the stage.
    - Patients with stage IA melanoma have a 5-year survival expectancy of 99%.
    - Stage IV disease estimated 5-year survival rate was estimated to be about <10% before the advent of newer targeted therapies.
  - Treatments are determined by Breslow depth and tumor stage and can include wide local excision, Mohs surgery, immunotherapy (i.e. PD-1 and CTLA-4 inhibitors) and BRAF inhibitors.
  - The discovery of newer targeted agents and immune checkpoint inhibitors has led to increased survival rates for both stage III and IV melanomas over the past decade!
- USMLE Board Review Pearls
  - Melanoma is one of the most common deadly diseases seen in dermatology. Melanoma sounds like a benign disease, so sometimes it is referred to as "malignant melanoma." Melanoma can affect any part of the body that has melanocytes such as the uveal tract of the eye or leptomeninges, so it is sometimes further referred to as "cutaneous malignant melanoma."
  - Look for an obviously different or "ugly-duckling" skin lesion in a patient with a history of a lighter skin tone and a history of multiple acquired and dysplastic melanocytic nevi.
  - Breslow depth correlates with risk of metastasis.
  - ALM has the highest prevalence in patients with darker skin tones (Bob Marley died of ALM at 36 years old).
  - BRAF is a key mutation in melanoma.
  - Lesions confined to the skin, that are thin and non-ulcerated, are usually treated with wide local excision only, and metastatic melanoma is treated with systemic therapies such as immunotherapy, BRAF inhibitors and MEK inhibitors. Thicker lesions or lesions with ulceration usually require a sentinel lymph node biopsy. Consult the AJCC (American Joint Committee on Cancer) staging system for melanoma for further information.
  - Sentinel lymph node biopsy is used for staging and prognosis but does not directly impact survival.
  - Know the classic features/morphology of the following types of melanoma: superficial spreading, nodular, ALM, lentigo maligna, and amelanotic melanoma (difficult to identify, usually will present as new/erythematous/growing lesion without clinical pigmentation).

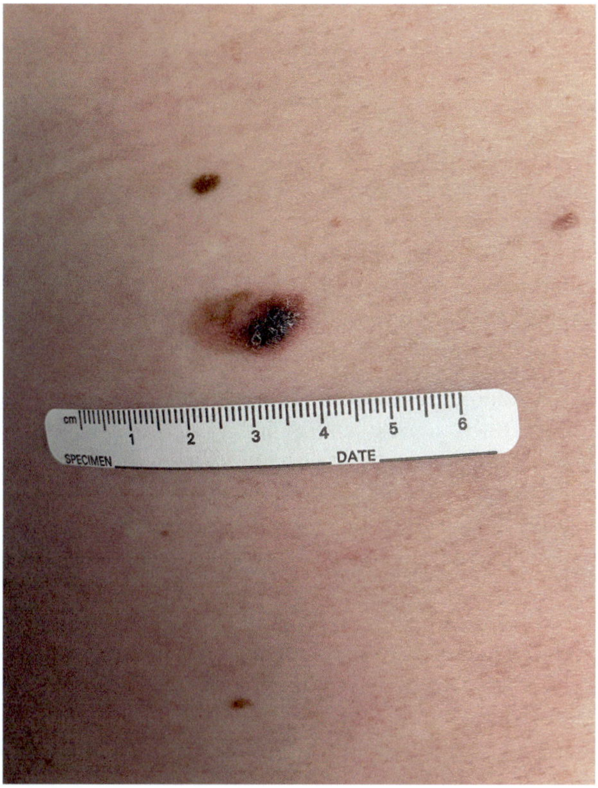

58. Melasma

- Morphology/clinical features
  - Light to dark brown patches with irregular borders.
- Distribution
  - Face.
    - Occasionally seen on the forearms.
    - Rarely seen on the upper chest.
- Etiology/pathogenesis
  - Exact pathogenesis unknown but theorized to be secondary to hyperfunctional melanocytes from triggers such as hormones or UV radiation.
    - Explains why melasma is also referred to as the "mask of pregnancy."
- Internal sequelae/comorbidities
  - None.

- Laboratory testing
  - None.
- Treatments/prognosis
  - Difficult to treat and completely cure!
  - The most important treatment for any melasma patient is strict photoprotection and sun avoidance.
  - Can lighten the hyperpigmentation with hydroquinone, tretinoin, and PO tranexamic acid (250 mg BID for 8–12 weeks). In clinical practice, tranexamic acid is dispensed at 650 mg, which can be split into 325 mg tablets and taken twice a day.
    - Triple-combination topical therapy with hydroquinone + corticosteroid + retinoid is more effective than topical hydroquinone alone.
    - Tranexamic acid may increase hypercoagulability, so must ask patients about history of smoking, OCP use, or other hypercoagulable states (cancer, history of blood clots) before prescribing.
- USMLE Board Review Pearls
  - Look for a female patient with dark brown irregular symmetric patches on the forehead or cheeks. The patient will be asymptomatic.
  - This is an acquired hyperpigmentary disorder that is commonly seen in pregnancy due to hormonal imbalances.
  - Besides melasma, other skin changes in pregnancy include linea nigra, nipple hyperpigmentation, and striae.
  - Oral contraceptive use can also lead to melasma.
  - The number 1 most important treatment principle with any melasma patient is strict photoprotection.

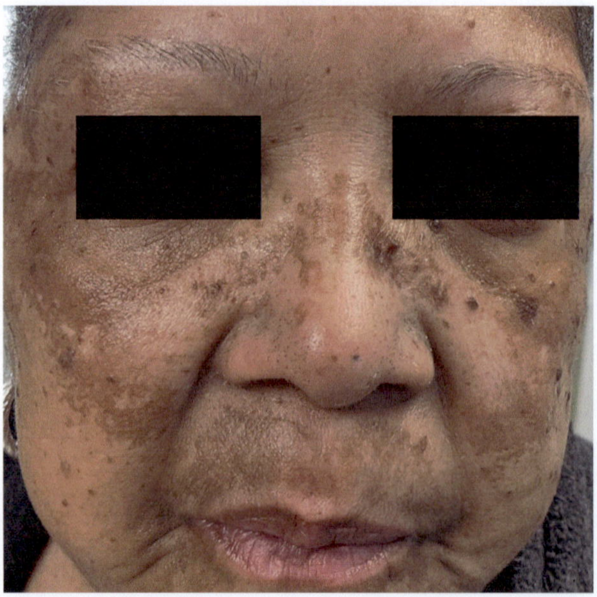

59. Merkel cell carcinoma (MCC)

- Morphology/clinical features
  - Pink to red/violaceous papulonodule.
- Distribution
  - Favors head and neck.
- Etiology/pathogenesis
  - UV radiation and Merkel cell polyomavirus (MCPyV).
    - 20% of lesions are MCPyV negative.
- Internal sequelae/comorbidities
  - Metastasis to internal organs.
- Laboratory testing
  - None.
- Treatments/prognosis.
  - Five-year overall survival was 50% (local disease), 35% (nodal disease), and 15% (distant disease) prior to the introduction of immunotherapy.
  - Sentinel lymph node positivity at the time of diagnosis is estimated to be about 35%.
- USMLE Board Review Pearls
  - Merkel cell carcinoma is the deadliest skin cancer.
  - Look for a large, prominent red/violaceous papulonodule on the scalp or face of an elderly patient. Ulceration may be present.
  - Merkel cells are part of normal skin anatomy/physiology (located in the superficial dermis), are found in high concentrations on the fingertips, and are responsible for detecting pressure and deep static touch (i.e., shapes and edges).
  - A Merkel cell is a type of large, myelinated fiber that adapts slowly to stimuli.
  - There are three FDA-approved immune checkpoint inhibitor medications to treat MCC: avelumab, pembrolizumab, and retifanlimab.
  - Patients negative for MCPyV have more aggressive tumors (i.e., MCPvY positivity is a better prognosis).
  - Negative immunostaining for thyroid transcription factor 1 (TTF-1) on histology helps differentiate MCC from cutaneous metastases of other small cell carcinomas.

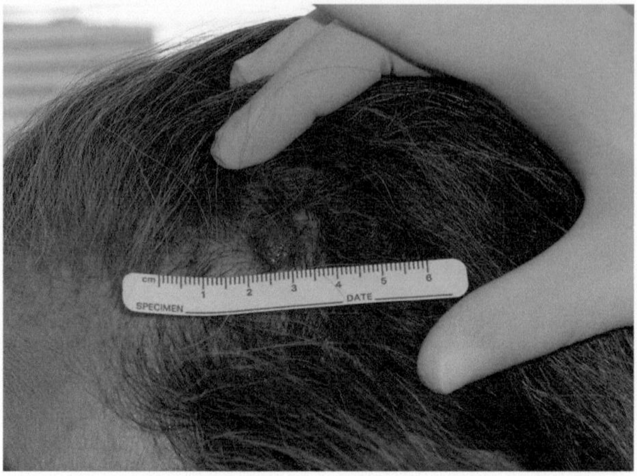

60. Miliaria

- Morphology/clinical features
  - Crystallina—nonpruritic clear, fragile vesicles.
  - Rubra—pruritic, erythematous, papules (may see pustules).
  - Profunda—nonpruritic, small white papules.
- Distribution
  - Face, trunk, and extremities.
    - Any areas of occlusion.
- Etiology/pathogenesis
  - Sweat retention within eccrine ducts from eccrine duct obstruction.
  - Seen in hot, humid climates or neonates (from over-swaddling or warming inside an incubator).
- Internal sequelae/comorbidities
  - None.
- Laboratory testing
  - None.
- Treatments/prognosis
  - Self-resolving.
  - Prevent by avoidance of overheating or by avoidance of excessive swaddling/occlusion.
- USMLE Board Review Pearls
  - Commonly known as "heat rash."

- Look for an infant with tiny, superficial clear vesicles on the neck and trunk. They will likely have a history of being swaddled.
- Affects up to 15% of newborns and not present at birth.
- Know where the blockage occurs in the sweat duct.
  - Crystallina—stratum corneum.
  - Rubra—mid-epidermis.
  - Profunda—dermal–epidermal junction.
- Do not confuse miliaria with malaria (infectious disease), milia (cyst), or apocrine miliaria (Fox–Fordyce disease).
- Treatment of choice is the prevention of overheating/occlusion but can use topical corticosteroids if severe symptoms are present.

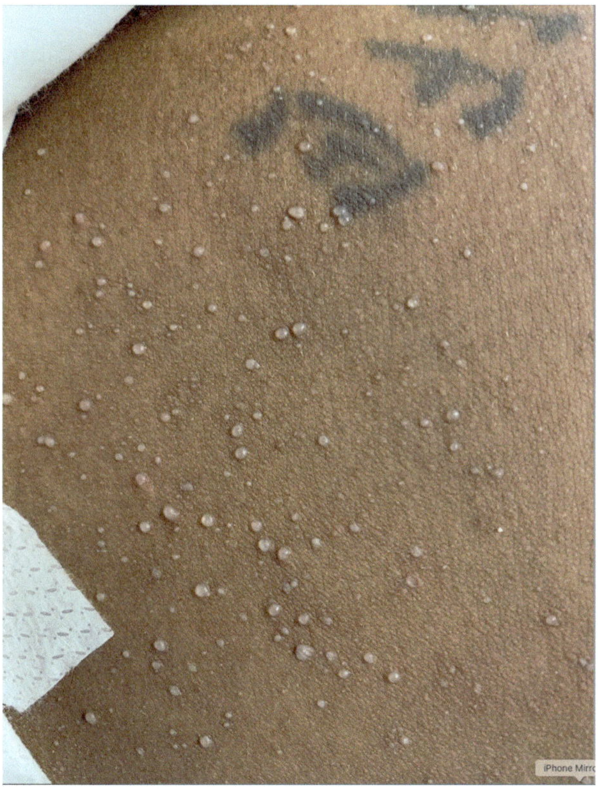

61. Molluscum contagiosum

- Morphology/clinical features
  - Well-demarcated umbilicated pink papules.

- Distribution
  - Intertriginous areas, trunk, extremities, and buttocks.
  - Genitals in sexually transmitted cases.
- Etiology/pathogenesis
  - Caused by a poxvirus.
- Internal sequelae/comorbidities
  - None.
- Laboratory testing
  - None.
- Treatments/prognosis
  - Will self-resolve with time but risk of spreading to self and others if not treated.
  - Can treat with physical modalities such as curettage and cryosurgery.
  - There are two FDA-approved topical medications: Berdazimer topical gel 10.3% and Ycanth© (cantharidin).
- USMLE Board Review Pearls
  - Look for small, numerous dome-shaped shiny umbilicated papules on the trunk or extremities of a child or on the genitals of a sexually active adult.
  - Poxvirus is an enveloped double-stranded linear DNA virus.
  - Spread by direct skin-to-skin contact (sexual intercourse, sports [wrestling]).
  - Biopsy will show large intracytoplasmic inclusion bodies called Henderson–Patterson bodies.
  - Lesions will resolve spontaneously in children but if left untreated will spread to self and others. First-line therapy for a few isolated lesions is destruction including curettage or cryosurgery.

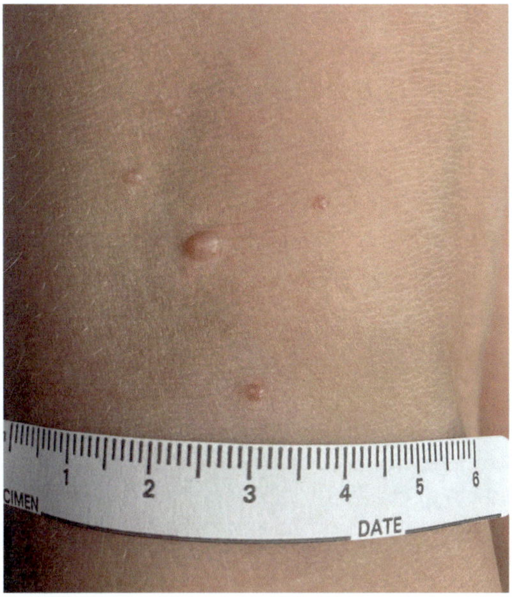

62. Morphea

- Morphology/clinical features
  - Begins as erythematous to violaceous patch that evolves into indurated, ivory plaque that is often anhidrotic or alopecic.
    - This is the presentation of plaque-type morphea, which is the most common form overall.
- Distribution
  - Most common on the trunk and extremities.
- Etiology/pathogenesis
  - Exact pathogenesis unknown but thought to be related to vascular damage, T-cell proliferation, and increase in connective tissue production by fibroblasts.
  - Linear morphea in children and adults with generalized morphea is a/w positive ANA.
- Internal sequelae/comorbidities
  - Linear morphea can lead to joint contractures, undergrowth of limbs, and joint deformity.

  - Parry–Romberg syndrome (a.k.a. progressive hemifacial atrophy) is a head/neck subtype of linear morphea that may be a/w epilepsy, exophthalmos, headaches, or trigeminal neuralgia.
  - Generalized morphea may lead to respiratory impairment due to constrictive effects of the tight skin on the chest.

- Laboratory testing
  - All forms have positive anti-topoisomerase II antibodies (75% overall, even higher in generalized morphea).

- Treatments/prognosis
  - You do not need to treat a single plaque of morphea if there is no functional or aesthetic impairment. Plaque-type morphea will soften and self-resolve over a few years (although PIH may persist).
  - Topical corticosteroids or intralesional steroids can be used.
  - The treatment of choice for moderate to severe morphea (i.e., generalized morphea) is methotrexate in combination with systemic steroids for a few months.

- USMLE Board Review Pearls
  - Look for an indurated, well-demarcated ivory white plaque with a violaceous rim. The patient will complain the area feels "hard" or "stiff."
  - Morphea lacks lack anti-Scl70 (Topo I) and anti-centromere antibodies.
    - Scleroderma is positive for these antibodies.
    - Morphea can be thought of as "localized scleroderma" = localized/limited skin thickening that does not affect any internal organs.
  - Linear and generalized morphea are more likely to be ANA positive compared to other forms of morphea.
  - Linear morphea is often positive for ssDNA antibodies. Linear morphea is the most common type in children and requires therapy to prevent joint contractures including a referral to physical therapy.
  - "En coup de sabre" is a subtype of linear head and neck morphea. Patients will present with an indented appearance on the forehead/scalp. These patients (along with Parry–Romberg syndrome patients) require regular eye exams by ophthalmology. Neurology referral should also be considered.

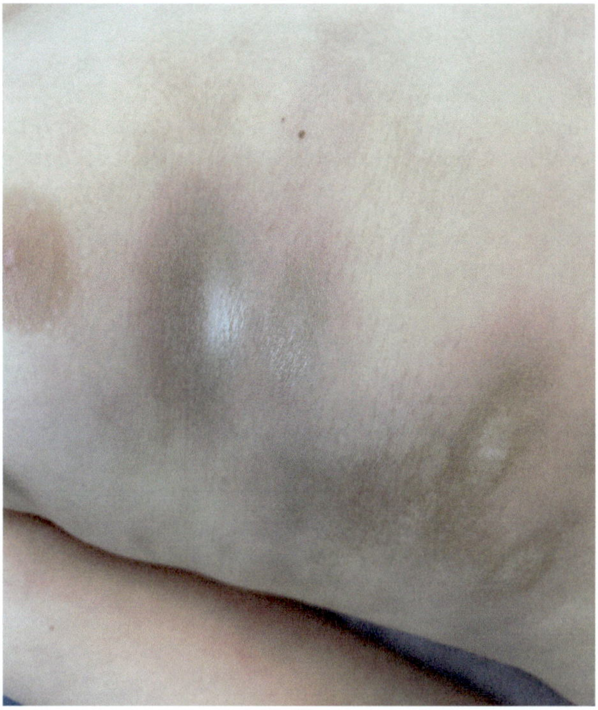

63. Mycosis fungoides (MF, cutaneous T-cell lymphoma)

- Morphology/clinical features/distribution
  - Patch stage—irregular erythematous patches with fine scale with prominent involvement of the "double covered areas" (non-sun-exposed areas like the buttocks, which is covered by both the underwear and pants).
  - Plaque stage—well-demarcated dull-red to erythematous plaques.
  - Tumor stage—rapidly growing erythematous nodules with ulceration arising in the background of patch or plaque stage MF.
- Etiology/pathogenesis
  - Unknown but thought to be secondary to a mixture of genetic, environmental, and immunologic factors.
  - This is a T-cell-driven skin lymphoma.
- Internal sequelae/comorbidities
  - Extracutaneous disease may develop and is correlated with the extent of skin disease.
    - Usually starts in regional lymph nodes and rarely may progress to visceral involvement.

- Laboratory testing
  - The neoplastic cells in MF have a CD3+, CD4+, CD8− immunophenotype.
  - The diagnosis is confirmed with a skin biopsy but it may take many years and many skin biopsies to confirm the diagnosis due to the indolent nature of the disease.
    - T-cell gene rearrangement may be used to aid in the diagnosis of MF but a false positive may occur with other conditions such as eczema.
    - This test needs to be interpreted in the appropriate clinicopathological context.
- Treatments/prognosis
  - Patch stage MF has an excellent prognosis, and survival rate is nearly identical to age, race, and sex-matched controls.
  - Skin-directed therapies include topical or intralesional steroids, phototherapy, radiotherapy, and topical mechlorethamine.
  - Oral therapies include retinoids, histone deacetylase inhibitors, and mogamulizumab.
  - If there is lymph node or visceral involvement, patients will need management by an oncologist.
- USMLE Board Review Pearls
  - Look for erythematous plaques with fine scale in sun-protected areas. The exam question will usually show a picture of the patients' lower back and buttocks covered in characteristic lesions.
  - Mycosis fungoides is not a fungus but the plaques sometimes resemble tinea corporis because of their irregular, wavy borders.
  - This disease is chronic, smoldering, and more common in men.
  - Lesions begin as patches that progress to plaques and then skin tumors.
  - The diagnosis is made by a combination of clinical findings, histopathology, and immunophenotyping.
  - MF should be highly considered in any "eczema" or "atopic dermatitis" patient who is refractory to systemic therapy like dupilumab.
  - First-line skin-directed therapy is phototherapy and topical steroids. Further treatment options include chemotherapy, oral retinoids (bexarotene), monoclonal antibodies (mogamulizumab), and IFN-α.

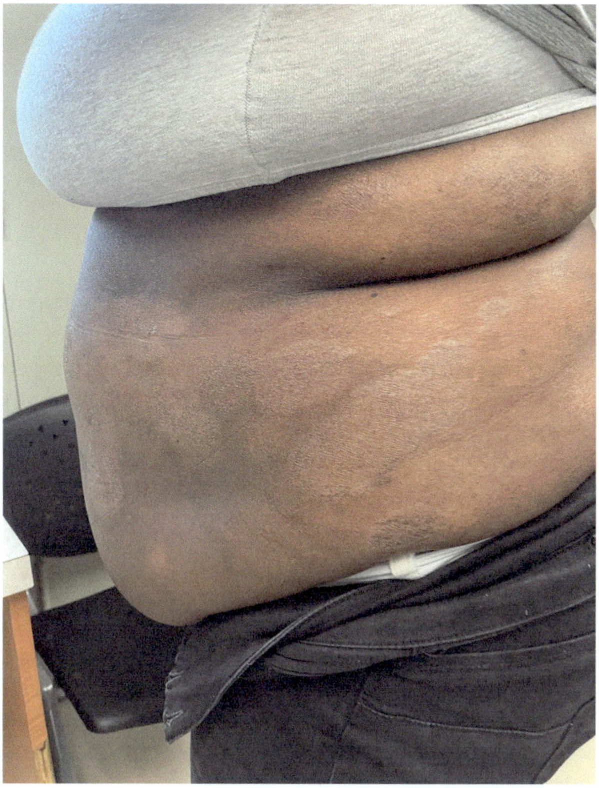

64. Nail diseases

This list is not comprehensive but represents some of the most high-yield nail diseases seen in clinical practice and on exams.

- **Beau's lines** are linear indentations in the nail plate usually due to mechanical trauma to the nail fold, skin disease of the nail fold, systemic illness, or severe stress.
- **Clubbing** of the nails/distal fingertips is soft tissue overgrowth, leading to a large and curved nail plate that is most commonly due to pulmonary disease.
- **Digital myxoid cyst** is a bluish/translucent, soft papule near the proximal nail fold that is formed from an outpouching of the DIP joint space.
- **Green nail syndrome** is characterized by green staining of the nail plate due to pyocyanin from a *Pseudomonas* infection.
- **Habit-tic deformity/median canaliform dystrophy** is a central linear, longitudinal depression/dystrophy in the nail plate from repetitive manipulation and picking. Median canaliform dystrophy is a subtype of habit-tic deformity characterized by a central depression with a branching, "fir-tree" morphology.

- **Half and half nails/Lindsay's nails** is an apparent leukonychia (white nail bed edema that fades with pressure) involving half of the nail bed that is associated with renal disease.
- **Koilonychia** is a spoon nail (concavity of the nail plate) that is normal in kids but in adults may be associated with iron deficiency.
- **Onychocryptosis** is the medical term for an ingrown toenail.
- **Onychogryphosis,** also known as Ram's horn nail, is a large, thickened, yellowish, hard, spiraled, and curved nail that grows out like a horn or claw due to neglect.
- **Onychomadesis** is nail splitting and nail dystrophy of the proximal nail fold commonly seen after *Coxsackievirus* infection (hand–foot–mouth disease).
- **Paronychia** is an infection of the nail fold that is caused by *staph* or *strep* in acute cases and *Candida* in chronic cases characterized by inflammation of the nail fold.
- **Pitting** of the nail plate can be seen in psoriasis and alopecia areata (where the pits are geometric and grid-like).
- **Psoriasis** of the nail plate is characterized by random nail pits, "oil spots" on the nail bed and onycholysis.
- **Splinter hemorrhages** are broken blood vessels that appear as red/brown lines in the nail bed due to trauma (distal hemorrhages) or in rare cases systemic diseases (proximal hemorrhages) due to infective endocarditis, vasculitis, or clotting disorders.
- **Subungual exostosis** is a rock-hard bony outgrowth from under the nail usually due to trauma that is most commonly on the great toe. First step in management is to obtain an X-ray.
- **Terry's nails** is an apparent leukonychia (white nail bed edema that fades with pressure) involving most of the nail bed that is associated with liver disease.
- **Trachyonychia** or "sandpaper nails" are nails that appear brittle and roughened with diffuse longitudinal ridging and can be accompanied by pitting and loss of sheen/luster that is due to lichen planus, alopecia areata, or other autoimmune diseases. Lichen planus can cause 20 nail dystrophy.
- **Yellow nail syndrome** is characterized by yellow-colored thickening/curved nails with absent cuticle and is associated with lymphedema, pleural effusions, and bronchiectasis.

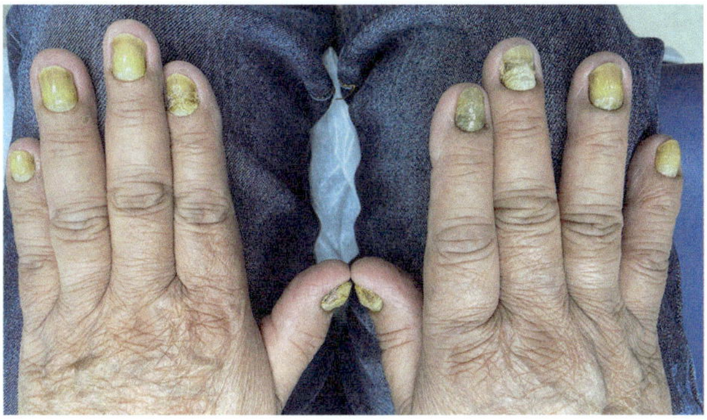

65. Necrobiosis lipodica (NLD)

- Morphology/clinical features
  - Classically presents as multiple yellowish atrophic plaques with noticeable telangiectasis surrounded by a peripheral erythematous-to-violaceous rim.
  - Lesions begin as firm, red papules.
  - Minor trauma results in ulceration.
- Distribution
  - Pretibial region.
    - NLD is practically never seen on other parts of the body besides this area, even though textbooks will mention that it is possible to see it in other areas of the body.
- Etiology/pathogenesis
  - Unknown but thought to be secondary to immunologically mediated vascular compromise and macroangiopathic vascular changes in diabetes patients.
- Internal sequelae/comorbidities
  - Only 0.03% of diabetics will develop NLD, but by some estimates, 60% of patients with NLD have diabetes.
    - Simply put, most diabetic patients will walk into your office without NLD, but if a patient has NLD, then they will very likely have diabetes or glucose intolerance.
- Laboratory testing
  - None.
- Treatments/prognosis

  - No effective treatments exist or have been proven in large, double-blinded placebo-controlled studies.
  - Many dermatologists will try topical corticosteroids (under occlusion), intralesional corticosteroids, or topical calcineurin inhibitors.
- USMLE Board Review Pearls
  - Look for atrophic red-brown-yellowish annular plaques on the pretibial skin with telangiectasias.
  - Screen for diabetes if a patient presents with NLD but has no history of diabetes.
  - These lesions may ulcerate (even with minor trauma).
  - Control of blood glucose does not impact disease course or outcome.
  - Rarely undergoes spontaneous remission.
  - If a patient has a new or changing lesion in an area of long-standing ulceration in NLD, need to biopsy to rule out SCC.

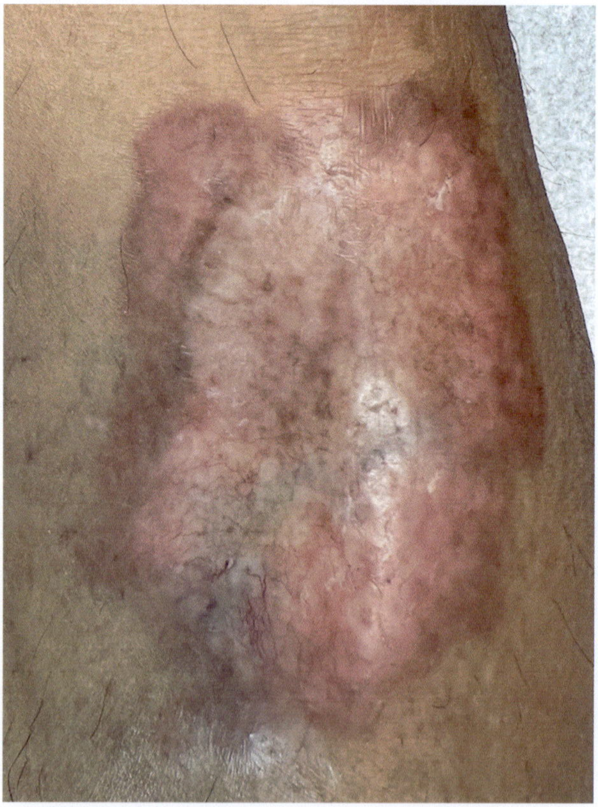

66. Nevus of Ota/Ito

- Morphology/clinical features/distribution
  - Ota = blue-gray patch in the periorbital region.
    - The O in Ota looks like an eye.
    - 60% will have scleral involvement.
  - Ito = blue-gray patch in the shoulder region.
- Etiology/pathogenesis
  - Dermal melanocytosis
    - Dermal melanocytes fail to migrate superiorly to dermoepidermal junction.
  - The blue color is due to the "Tyndall effect."
    - Blue wavelengths are reflected from the deeper melanin in the skin.
    - This phenomenon also partially explains why the sky is blue.
- Internal sequelae/comorbidities
  - 10% of patients with Nevus of Ota may develop glaucoma.
- Laboratory testing
  - None.
- Treatments/prognosis
  - Treatment of choice is ruby, alexandrite, or Nd:YAG laser.
- USMLE Board Review Pearls
  - Look for blue-gray patch of skin around the eye or around the shoulder.
  - Patients with Nevus of Ota should have an ophthalmology referral to screen for glaucoma.
  - Treatment of choice is ruby laser.
  - Will not fade on its own.

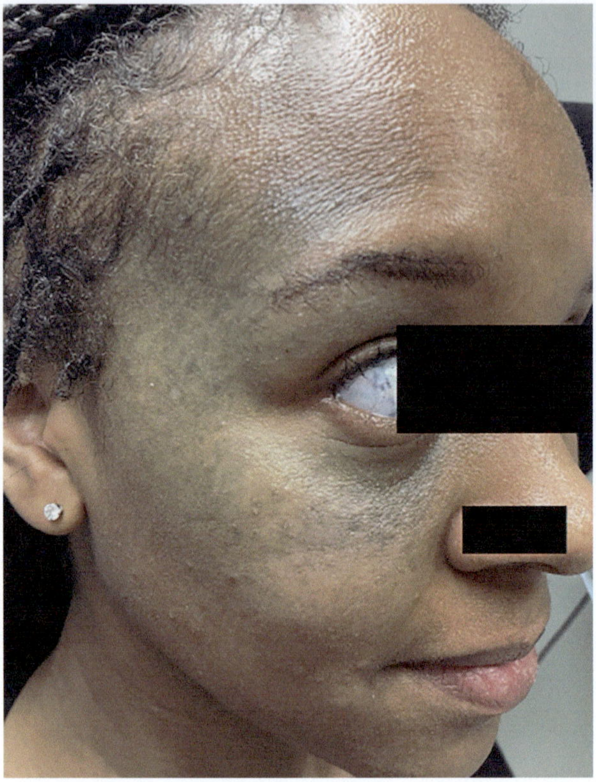

67. Pellagra

- Morphology/clinical features/distribution
  - Casal's necklace = well-demarcated hyperpigmented patch around the neck.
  - Photodistributed erythema that may have a "shellac"-like appearance.
  - Cheilitis and glossitis.
  - Painful fissures of the palms and soles.
- Etiology/pathogenesis
  - Due to a vitamin B_3 (niacin) deficiency.
- Internal sequelae/comorbidities
  - Can see peripheral neuropathy, diarrhea, nausea, dementia, and esophagitis.
- Laboratory testing
  - Check vitamin B_3 level.

  - Causes include Hartnup disease, alcoholism, carcinoid syndrome, medications (isoniazid, 5-FU, azathioprine), anorexia, and malabsorption syndromes.

- Treatments/prognosis
  - Nicotinamide 300 mg/day PO (in divided doses) x 3–4 weeks, then maintenance of niacin (for adult patients).
- USMLE Board Review Pearls
  - Look for a patient with a hyperpigmented well-demarcated patch around the neck in a "necklace" distribution with erythema and scaling of the tongue and lips as well as photodistributed redness. The patient will likely also present with diarrhea and/or altered mental status.
  - Due to a deficiency in vitamin B_3.
    - On exams, look for Hartnup disease or carcinoid syndrome as a cause.
      - Hartnup disease is an AR condition that is caused by defective amino acid transport causing low niacin levels from malabsorption of tryptophan.
      - Patients with carcinoid syndrome develop pellagra because tryptophan is metabolized by serotonin, which is increased in carcinoid syndrome.
  - The classic presentation of pellagra is the 4 Ds.
    - Diarrhea, dementia, dermatitis, and death.

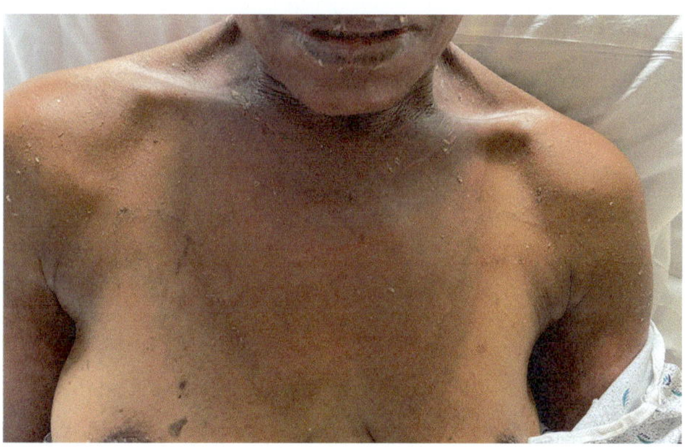

68. Pemphigus foliaceus

- Morphology/clinical features
  - Crusted erosions on an erythematous base with loose "cornflake"-like scale.

  - "Cornflake" scale is due to very fragile/superficial bullae that easily rupture.
  - No mucosal involvement.
- Distribution
  - Favors seborrheic distribution that includes face, scalp, and upper trunk.
- Etiology/pathogenesis
  - This is an autoimmune blistering disease that is caused by autoantibodies to desmoglein 1 (desmogleins are a part of desmosomes that are cell-to-cell adhesion molecules that provide structural support via intermediate filament interactions).
- Internal sequelae/comorbidities
  - None.
- Laboratory testing
  - Guinea pig esophagus is the substrate of choice when performing an indirect immunofluorescence with the patient's serum.
- Treatments/prognosis
  - Systemic steroids and topical corticosteroids.
  - Not severely ill and almost no risk of mortality.
- USMLE Board Review Pearls
  - Look for a patient with widespread erythematous plaques with loose, flaking scale on the upper chest, back, face, and scalp. The patient will not appear ill, and intact blisters will unlikely be present.
  - There is no mucosal involvement.
  - Drug-induced pemphigus usually presents with a pemphigus foliaceus-like presentation.
    - Common drugs include penicillamine, ACEi, and ARBs.
  - Caused by autoantibodies to desmoglein 1.
    - Desmoglein 1 is also the target in staph scaled skin syndrome (SSSS) from the production of exfoliative toxin.

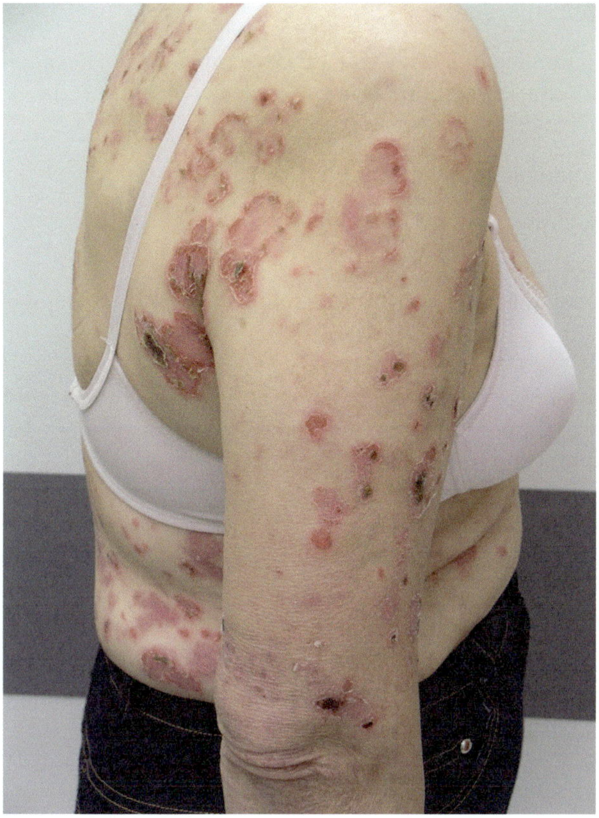

69. Pemphigus vulgaris

- Morphology/clinical features
  - Painful oral erosions with irregular borders
    - Other mucosal sites include esophagus, nasal mucosa, and mucosa of genitals and anus.
    - The scalp is frequently involved.
    - The painful oral erosions are sometimes referred to as "SJS mouth."
  - Flaccid bullae on the skin
    - These easily erupt and form crusted lesions.
    - Positive Nikolsky sign and Asboe–Hansen sign.
- Distribution
  - Oral erosions most commonly seen on buccal and palatine mucosal.

- Etiology/pathogenesis
  - Autoimmune blistering disease with antibodies to desmoglein 3 (Dsg3).
- Internal sequelae/comorbidities
  - May be a/w other autoimmune diseases such as myasthenia gravis and autoimmune thyroiditis.
- Laboratory testing
  - ELISA for Dsg3.
  - DIF demonstrates cell-surface "chicken-wire" staining with IgG.
- Treatments/prognosis
  - Dermatology emergency! Nearly all patients who are misdiagnosed and not treated properly will die from widespread skin denudation, leading to fluid loss and infection.
  - First line is PO steroids (1 mg/kg per day), then switch to a nonsteroidal immunosuppressive agent.
  - Rituximab is FDA approved for the treatment of pemphigus vulgaris. The 2020 International Consensus Guidelines recommend rituximab plus systemic corticosteroids as first-line therapy for moderate to severe pemphigus vulgaris.
    - Hepatitis B serologies need to be checked before starting this medication.
- USMLE Board Review Pearls
  - Look for flaccid bullae leading to crusted skin lesions and painful oral erosions in a patient who is in the 40s–60s age range.
    - Patients will bullous pemphigoid are usually older in their 60s–70s.
  - Due to autoantibodies to Dsg3 (mucosal-dominant pemphigus) or both Dsg1 and Dsg3 (mucocutaneous pemphigus).
  - Always need to consider this diagnosis in an elderly patient with genital erosions.
  - Pemphigus vulgaris bleeds as opposed to pemphigus foliaceus.
  - On the skin, erosions are more commonly seen than tense bullae because the blisters easily rupture.
    - This is opposite to bullous pemphigoid where tense blisters are more commonly seen than crusted/unroofed lesions.
    - This is because the location of the split in pemphigus vulgaris is more superficial (intraepidermal), whereas the split in bullous pemphigoid is deeper (basement membrane zone).
      - The more superficial the split in the skin—the more flaccid and weaker the resulting blister will be.

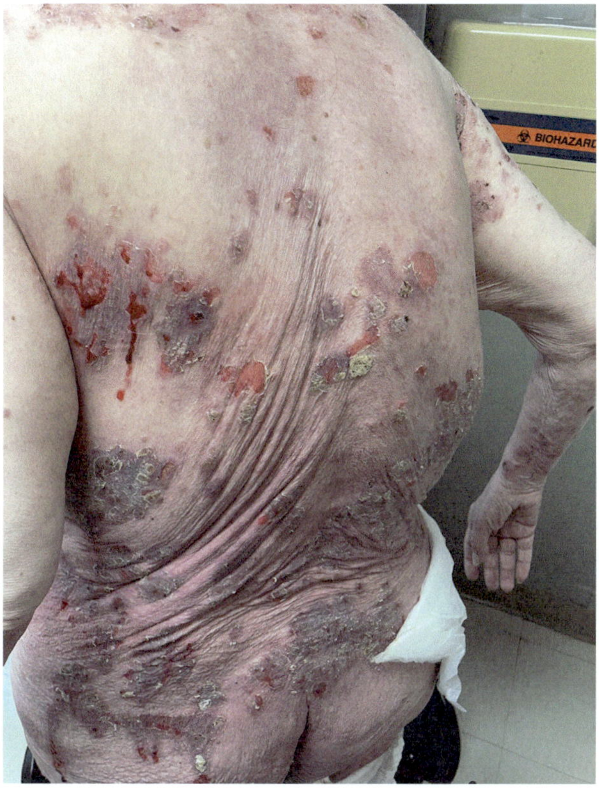

70. Periorificial dermatitis

- Morphology/clinical features
  - Clusters of small monomorphic pinpoint erythematous to pink pinpoint papules and pustules.
  - Patients usually complain of burning as opposed to itching.
- Distribution
  - Periorbital region, periocular region, and perioral region.
- Etiology/pathogenesis
  - Unknown etiology but thought to be exacerbated or caused by facial cosmetics/moisturizers and fluorinated steroids.

- Internal sequelae/comorbidities
  - None.
- Laboratory testing
  - None.
- Treatments/prognosis
  - Avoid cosmetics, moisturizers, and topical steroids on or around the area.
  - Oral tetracyclines and topical clindamycin, topical metronidazole.
  - Isotretinoin can be used in recalcitrant cases.
- USMLE Board Review Pearls
  - Look for a patient with identical appearing pink to red clustered papules around the mouth, nares, or eyes. The papules may involve all or only one of these areas. The patient will likely have a history of using facial cosmetics/moisturizers or steroid use in the area.
  - Do not misdiagnose this condition as eczema in the periorbital distribution.
  - Commonly affects young women in 20–30s but children can be affected too.
  - This is an inflammatory condition of the face that some consider a variant of rosacea.
  - There is usually a zone of normal skin around the vermillion border when the condition involves the perioral region.
  - If the patient denies using any topical corticosteroids, a history of inhaled corticosteroids for asthma may be elicited from the patient and could be the cause of perioral dermatitis.

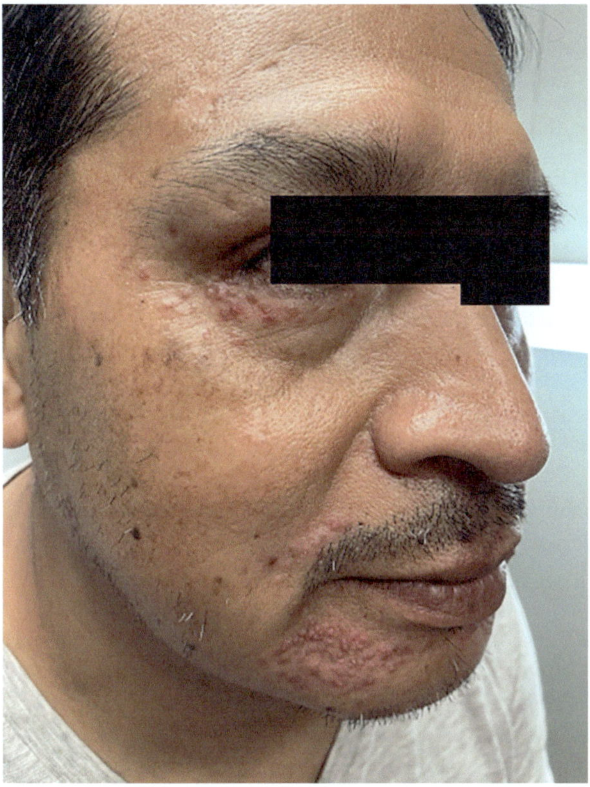

71. Phytophotodermatitis

- Morphology/clinical features
  - Acutely presents as **linear streaks** of erythema (with or without blistering), but patients usually present later with linear streaks of post-inflammatory hyperpigmentation.
    - A "splash" pattern of post-inflammatory hyperpigmentation may also be observed.
- Distribution
  - Hands and forearms most commonly seen.
    - Also can be observed on the trunk and lower extremities.
- Etiology/pathogenesis
  - A phototoxic reaction caused by a combination of a topical photosensitizing agent and sunlight (UVA radiation).

    - Common photosensitizers include citrus (lemon, lime, grapefruit), parsley, parsnips, celery, and hogweed.
  - A classic presentation is a bartender who is making margaritas or guacamole at an outdoor bar near a beach or pool.
    - In this scenario, lime juice is the photosensitizing agent.
- Internal sequelae/comorbidities
  - None.
- Laboratory testing
  - None.
- Treatments/prognosis
  - Prevention is the best treatment.
    - Counsel the patient on the etiology and to avoid photosensitizing triggers when exposed to sunlight.
- USMLE Board Review Pearls
  - Look for a bartender or college student with bizarre, nongeometric, linear dark brown streaks or patches on the hands and forearms. The patient will likely report a history of making guacamole or margaritas in the sun.
  - This is a phototoxic reaction (not an allergic contact dermatitis), so patients do not require a previous exposure and anyone can be affected.
  - The chemical name for the photosensitizing agent is furocoumarin, and the wavelength of light that is implicated in this process is 320–400 nm (UVA radiation).
  - The term "phytophotodermatitis" is used to emphasize that a combination of plants ("phyto-") plus light ("photo-") is required for this process.

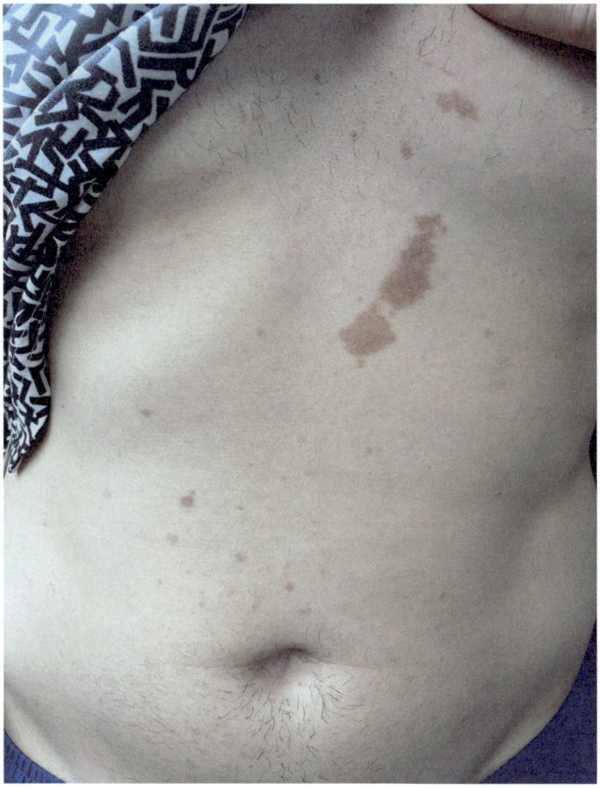

72. Pigmented purpuric dermatosis

- Morphology/clinical features
  - A group of disorders with hallmark findings of clustered petechial hemorrhages.
  - Schamberg's = brown/yellowish/erythematous macules and patches with pinpoint red petechial "cayenne pepper" spots.
  - Purpura annularis telangiectodes of Majocchi = annular patches with punctate red petechiae on the border.
  - Lichenoid dermatitis of Gougerot and Blum = combination of Schamberg's-like lesions and rust-colored lichenoid papules.
  - Eczematid-like purpura of Doucas and Kapetanakis = scaly, eczematous plaques with petechiae.
  - Lichen aureus = solitary golden or "rust-colored" patch.
- Distribution
  - Most commonly seen on lower extremities.

- Etiology/pathogenesis
  - Inflammation of the capillaries with resultant hemorrhage (capillaritis).
- Internal sequelae/comorbidities
  - None.
- Laboratory testing
  - None.
- Treatments/prognosis
  - Topical corticosteroids for pruritus.
  - Successful therapy with ascorbic acid (500 mg twice daily) plus rutoside (50 mg twice daily) has also been reported.
  - May self-resolve but could take months to years.

USMLE Board Review Pearls

- Look for erythematous/hyperpigmented patches on the lower extremities with pinpoint hemorrhages.
- These diseases have no systemic findings.
- The reason for the inflammation/capillaritis is unknown.
- May present on the lower extremities after vigorous physical activity in hot climates, where it is sometimes called "Golfer's vasculitis" or "Disney rash" (from walking long distances through theme parks in the hot Florida sun).

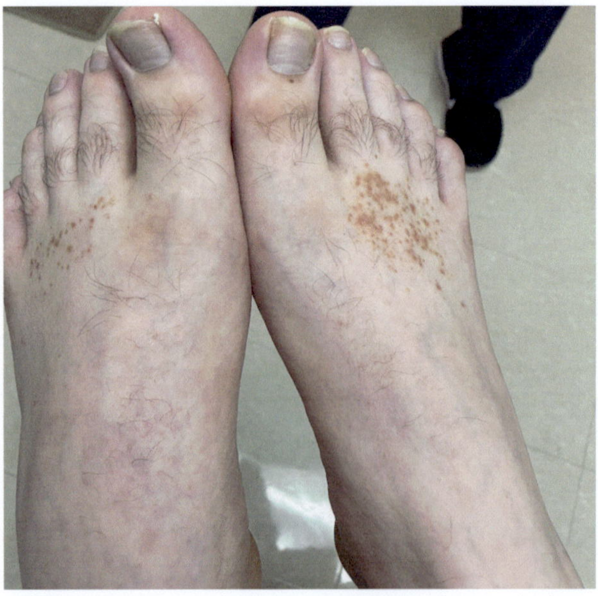

73. Pityriasis rosea

- Morphology/clinical features
  - Begins with a large, solitary erythematous/pink plaque (herald patch) with fine trailing scale on the trunk followed by an acute eruption of widespread smaller lesions with similar morphology, forming a characteristic "Christmas tree" pattern on the back.
- Distribution
  - Trunk and extremities
    - The herald patch is usually on the trunk.
- Etiology/pathogenesis
  - Exact pathogenesis unknown but considered to be a prototypical "paraviral exanthem" = skin rash associated with a possible viral infection or reactivation of a viral infection but without the ability to identify a specific infectious agent from the skin lesions.
- Internal sequelae/comorbidities
  - None.
- Laboratory testing
  - None.
    - Many dermatologists will get a rapid plasma reagin (RPR) test to rule out secondary syphilis when an adolescent or adult patient presents with pityriasis rosea as these eruptions can present similarly.
      - "When you think PR, check RPR."
- Treatments/prognosis
  - None, this eruption is often asymptomatic and self-limited.
  - Can use topical corticosteroids for pruritus.
  - About 2% of patients may get pityriasis rosea again.
- USMLE Board Review Pearls
  - Look for an acute eruption with one large lesion (herald patch) and numerous smaller similar lesions on the trunk. The papules and plaques are usually arranged following skin lines on the back, giving a "Christmas tree" pattern. The lesions will have fine trailing scale, and the smaller lesions will usually erupt days to weeks after the herald patch.
  - The etiology is unknown but is hypothesized to represent a viral reactivation of human herpesvirus 7 (HHV-7).
  - This is a clinical diagnosis but should have a low threshold to test the patient for secondary syphilis with an RPR test.

– The rash will self-resolve in 6–8 weeks without treatment but can give supportive therapy, including topical corticosteroids or anti-histamines for pruritus.

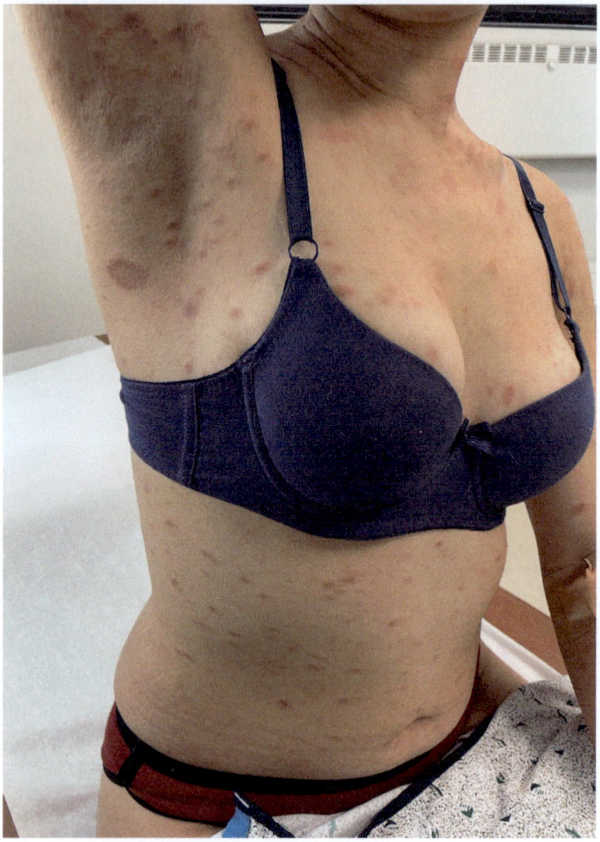

74. Pityriasis lichenoides (PLC/PLEVA)

- Morphology/clinical features

  – Recurrent crops of self-resolving lesions

    - Pityriasis lichenoides et varioliformis acuta (PLEVA) = acute form of pityriasis lichenoides characterized by scaly reddish-brown papules that evolve into crusted and necrotic lesions.

      – PLEVA is also known as Mucha–Habermann disease.
      – "Febrile ulceronecrotic Mucha–Habermann disease" is a distinctive variant of PLEVA/Mucha–Habermann disease.

  - Pityriasis lichenoides chronica (PLC) = chronic form of PLEVA that is characterized by scaly red/brown papules and plaques (some with a prominent "psoriasis like" central scale) that resolve with **hypopigmentation.**

- Distribution
  - Trunk, buttocks, and extremities.
- Etiology/pathogenesis
  - Unknown but postulated to be a T-cell lymphoproliferative disorder in response to a foreign antigen such as infection or medication.
- Internal sequelae/comorbidities
  - "Febrile ulceronecrotic Mucha–Habermann disease" is a rare PLEVA variant characterized by larger necrotic lesions, fever, constitutional symptoms, lymphadenopathy, arthritis, mucosal, pulmonary, and GI involvement.
    - a/w with increased TNF-α levels and 15% mortality rate.
- Laboratory testing
  - None.
- Treatments/prognosis
  - Start with tetracyclines or macrolide antibiotics.
    - Used for their anti-inflammatory effects but do not work well.
  - More severe cases require low-dose weekly methotrexate, but some dermatologists may choose to start right away with methotrexate as it is much more effective.
- USMLE Board Review Pearls
  - Look for multiple scaly brown-red papules with necrotic papules in PLEVA and look for multiple scaly red/brown papules in PLC along with hypopigmented macules (PLC heals with hypopigmentation, PLEVA has more necrotic papules in the acute presentation).
  - PLC can sometimes be thought of as "psoriasis in the wrong distribution."
    - Scaly erythematous papules involving areas where psoriasis is uncommon such as the antecubital fossa, popliteal fossa, forearms, and neck.
  - Diffuse distribution is the fastest to self-resolve while peripheral distribution is the slowest to self-resolve.
  - The T-cell infiltrate is predominantly CD8+ T-cells.

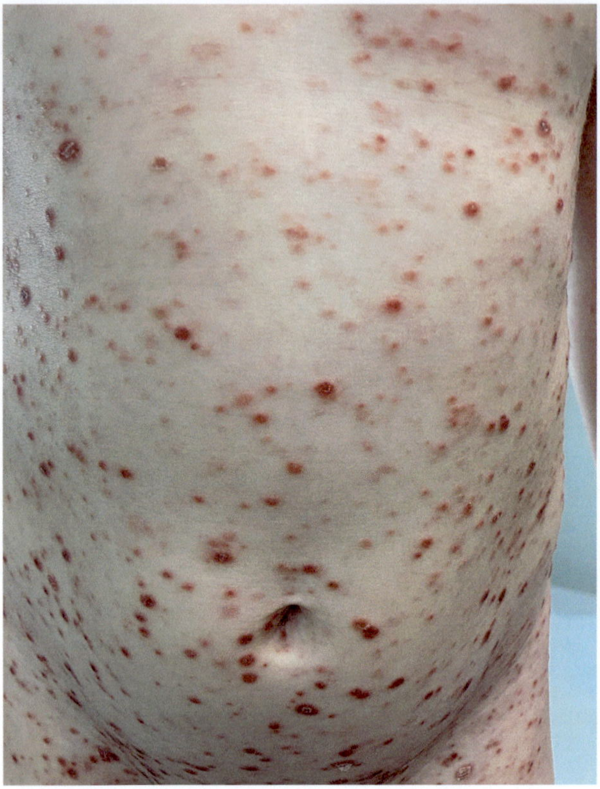

75. Polymorphous light eruption (PMLE)

- Morphology/clinical features
  - As the name implies clinical features are "polymorphous" and can be in the form of erythematous papules, vesicles, plaques, or pinpoint papules (more commonly seen in skin of color) associated with pruritus.
  - Arises 1–4 days after UV exposure, in some cases can be even sooner.
- Distribution
  - Sun-exposed areas such as dorsal hands, forearms, and upper V area of the neck and face.
- Etiology/pathogenesis
  - Unknown but thought to be secondary to delayed-type hypersensitivity reaction to UV radiation induced antigens in the skin.
- Internal sequelae/comorbidities
  - None.

- Laboratory testing
  - None.
- Treatments/prognosis
  - Photoprotection and counseling is first line.
  - Topical tacrolimus BID.
  - Phototherapy may be used to "harden" or "toughen" the skin in the early spring to reduce PMLE eruptions in the summer months.
- USMLE Board Review Pearls
  - This is the most common photosensitive dermatosis and by some estimates impacts up to 20% of Caucasian patients.
  - Look for a patient with a nonspecific eruption on sun-exposed areas associated with pruritus. Patients may present with mainly left-sided disease from long commutes in their car in the summer (the driver's left side is more exposed to UV radiation with the window down and from resting their arm on the open window sill of their car).
  - Most commonly occurs in spring and early summer in the Northern latitudes.
  - Arises 1–4 days after UV exposure and lesions last days to weeks.
  - Juvenile spring eruption is a variant seen mainly in pediatric and adolescent males.

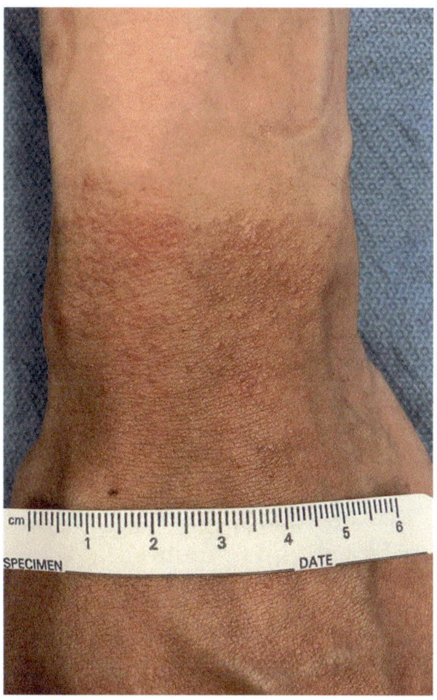

76. Pityriasis rubra pilaris (PRP)

- Morphology/clinical features
  - Classic adult type I is described as keratotic papules on an erythematous base ("nut-meg" grater papules) that coalesce into orange/salmon-colored plaques with classic "islands of sparing" (normal skin) in the plaques.
  - Orange/red waxy "carnauba wax" keratoderma and "sandal-like" keratoderma on the feet.
  - Thick, yellow-brown nails with subungual debris lacking pits.
  - Ectropion may be seen.
- Distribution
  - Classically begins on the head/neck region and progresses caudally.
- Etiology/pathogenesis
  - Unknown but thought to be an exaggerated secondary response to various triggers, including UV exposure, minor trauma to the skin, drugs, and vaccines.
  - Abnormal immunologic response to particular antigens may play a role.
- Internal sequelae/comorbidities
  - PRP rarely may present as a paraneoplastic disease.
  - PRP type VI is associated with HIV infection.
- Laboratory testing
  - None.
- Treatments/prognosis
  - Systemic retinoids are first-line therapy.
  - Classic adult type I form is typically self-limited, clearing within 3 years in nearly all patients.
- USMLE Board Review Pearls
  - Look for a patient with a widespread orange/salmon-colored rash with areas of normal skin along with thick, shiny, scaling plaques on the hands and feet with prominent scalp and facial involvement.
  - Type VI PRP is associated with HIV infection.
  - Mutations in *CARD14* have been implicated in PRP.
  - First-line therapy is acitretin (a retinoid).
  - Nail changes in PRP patient lack pits as opposed to nail changes in psoriasis patients that typically demonstrates pitting.

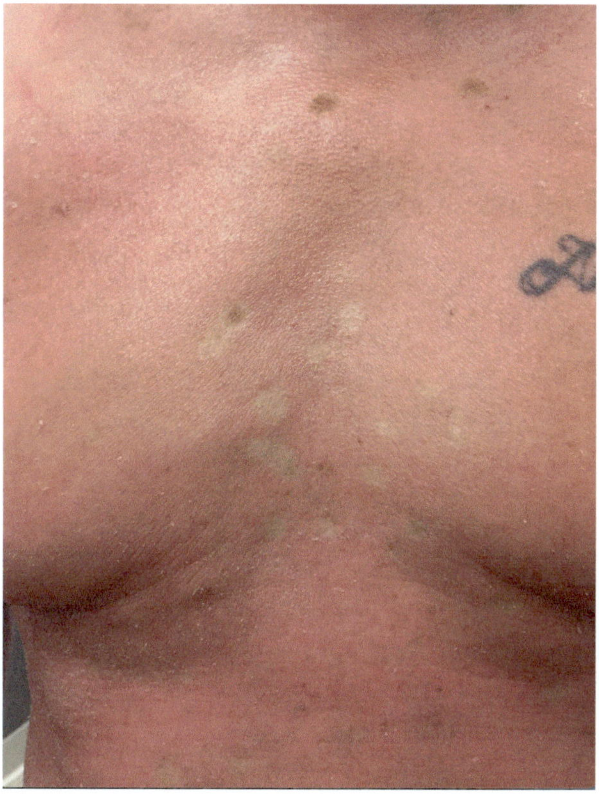

77. Prurigo nodularis

- Morphology/clinical features
  - Dome-shaped discrete, keratotic, skin-colored papules with thick central scale.
- Distribution
  - Any area of the skin that the patient can reach by scratching.
  - The mid-back is commonly spared because the patient cannot reach this area easily.
    - This is referred to as the "butterfly" sign.

- Etiology/pathogenesis
  - Prurigo nodularis is a sequela of chronic itch due to repetitive scratching or picking of the skin.
  - The development of an "itch-scratch" cycle can contribute to disease chronicity.
- Internal sequelae/comorbidities
  - Must evaluate the underlying reason for the pruritus.
    - This can include atopic dermatitis, xerosis, or a systemic disease, which manifests with pruritus.
      - Rarely malignancies can present with sudden, eruptive pruritus, leading to prurigo nodularis.
- Laboratory testing
  - None.
- Treatments/prognosis
  - There are two FDA-approved biologic therapies for prurigo nodularis:
    - Dupilumab (blocks IL-4 and IL-13).
    - Nemolizumab (blocks IL-31 receptor).
- USMLE Board Review Pearls
  - Look for multiple dome-shaped, skin-colored, papulonodules with central crust, excoriations, or erosions distributed on extensor extremities, trunk (but sparing the mid-back). The patient will complain of pruritus.
  - IL-31 is a key cytokine in the itch pathway.
  - One of the most common underlying cause of prurigo nodularis is atopic dermatitis.

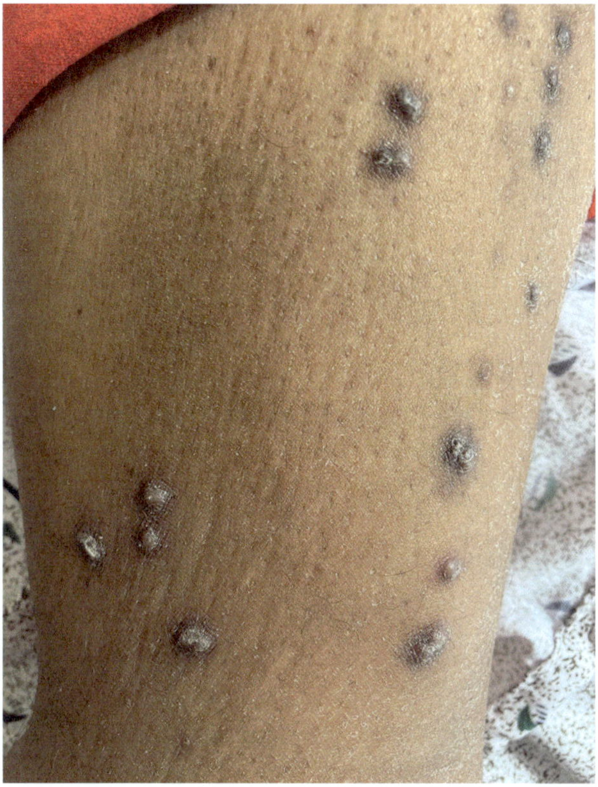

78. Psoriasis

- Morphology/clinical features
  - Plaque psoriasis/psoriasis vulgaris = well-demarcated pink/erythematous plaques and papules with thick, silvery white/ "micaceous scale."
  - Guttate (Latin for "rain drop") psoriasis = numerous widespread drop like papules and plaques on the trunk and extremities.
    - Usually associated with preceding group A *strep* infection.
  - Pustular psoriasis = erythematous/pink plaques studded with tiny pinpoint pustules.
  - Palmoplantar pustular psoriasis = pustules with yellow/brown macules localized on the palms and soles with well-demarcated pink/red scaling plaques.
  - Acrodermatitis continua of Hallopeau = a form of psoriasis limited to the distal fingertips characterized by pustules, pink/red scaling plaques that can lead to bony destruction.

- Distribution
  - Plaque psoriasis classically involves the scalp, elbow, knees, presacral area, genitals, and retroarticular area.
- Etiology/pathogenesis
  - Genetic component (*HLA-Cw6* allele most important).
  - Immune-mediated T-cell process driven by TNF-α, IL-17, and IL-23.
  - IL-23 is referred to as the "master cytokine" in the pathophysiology of psoriasis.
- Internal sequelae/comorbidities
  - Psoriatic arthritis in up to 30% of patients and is the most important comorbidity to recognize and manage.
  - Other important and recently recognized comorbidities include the risk of cardiovascular disease, metabolic disease, inflammatory bowel disease, malignancy, and mood disorders (depression and anxiety).
- Laboratory testing
  - None.
- Treatments/prognosis
  - Topical corticosteroids, topical calcineurin inhibitors, topical vitamin D analogs, topical tapinarof (aryl hydrocarbon receptor agonist), and topical roflumilast (PDE-4 inhibitor).
  - Apremilast (PDE-4 inhibitor), acitretin, methotrexate, cyclosporine, and deucravacitinib (TYK 2 inhibitor).
  - Phototherapy (NB-UVB and PUVA).
  - Biologics
    - **TNF-α inhibitors**: infliximab, etanercept, adalimumab, and certolizumab.
    - **IL-12/IL-23 inhibitor**: ustekinumab.
    - **IL-17 inhibitors**: secukinumab, ixekizumab, brodalumab (blocks receptor), and bimekizumab.
    - **IL-23 inhibitors**: tildrakizumab, risankizumab, and guselkumab.
    - **IL-36 receptor blocker**: spesolimab (FDA approved for generalized pustular psoriasis).
- USMLE Board Review Pearls
  - Look for well-demarcated pink/erythematous papules and plaques with thick white/silvery scale on the extensor surfaces (especially elbows and knees).

- Nail involvement is characterized by pitting, “oil spots” on the nail bed and distal lifting/separation of the nail plate from the nail bed (onycholysis).
- This is a T-cell immune-mediated inflammatory skin disease that can be seen in any age group.
- Medication triggers include β-blockers, lithium, and ACEi.
- 30% of patients develop psoriatic arthritis that typically impacts the small joints on the hands and is manifested by morning stiffness, joint pain, and swollen fingers/dactylitis a.k.a. “sausage digits.”
  - “Pencil-in-cup” deformity seen on X-ray.
  - Psoriatic arthritis is a seronegative spondyloarthritis.
- Treat localized disease or skin disease without arthritis with topical therapy and moderate/severe disease or any amount of skin disease with arthritis with systemic therapy (i.e., biologic therapy).
- Obtain a TB test (PPD or interferon-gamma release assay = Quantiferon Gold) and hepatitis B serologies before starting a biologic therapy.
- Brodalumab is an IL-17 receptor blocker while all of the other IL-17 agents block IL-17A or IL-17A and IL-17F.
- Etanercept is different from other anti-TNF agents in that it is a fusion protein (decoy receptor for TNF-α + IgG1 Fc).

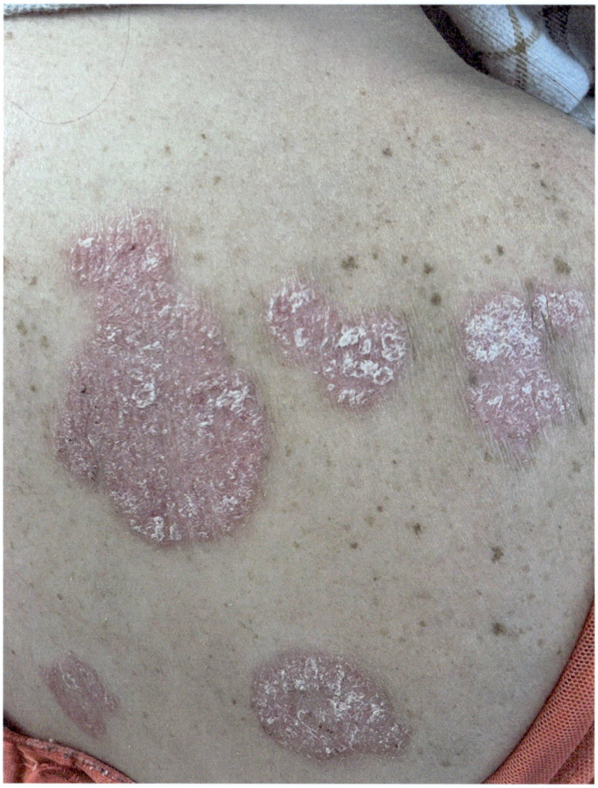

79. Pyoderma gangrenosum

- Morphology/clinical features
  - Classic form is described as a painful ulcer with undermined, overhanging irregular violaceous/gunmetal gray-colored border with a purulent and vegetative base.
  - Heals with cribriform scar.
- Distribution
  - Lower extremities (pretibial).
  - Can be seen on the dorsal foot.
- Etiology/pathogenesis
  - Idiopathic in 25–50% of cases but an unknown immunologic abnormality is suspected.
    - Increased activity of IL-1 is thought to play a central role.
  - Pathergy is seen in 20–30% of patients.
- Internal sequelae/comorbidities
  - Half of the cases have an associated systemic inflammatory disorder.
    - IBD is the most common.
    - Others include hematologic malignancy or inflammatory arthritis.
- Laboratory testing
  - Rule out underlying conditions.
    - Colonoscopy or stool studies.
    - Hematologic studies (such as CBC, peripheral smear, bone marrow biopsy).
- Treatments/prognosis
  - Every patient should be receiving good wound care.
  - Unfortunately, there is no specific or highly effective treatment for this condition.
  - Initial therapy is with systemic steroids.
    - Can then try and switch to a safer long-term systemic immunomodulatory agent such as a biologic (TNF-α inhibitor or IL12/23 inhibitor) or JAK inhibitor (tofacitinib, baricitinib).
  - Cyclosporine is another option.
- USMLE Board Review Pearls
  - Look for a very painful ulceration on the pretibial area with a violaceous, undermined border with a purulent base.

- Ulcers of pyoderma gangrenosum begin as papules or pustules but rapidly progress into frank ulcerations.
- Pathergy is a common feature of this disease.
  - Some patients are misdiagnosed or undiagnosed may have these ulcers debrided by a surgeon, which will cause them to become much worse (due to pathergy).
- Key systemic disease associations include inflammatory bowel disease, rheumatoid arthritis, and malignancy.
- Mild disease (small ulcers < 3 cm) can be treated with topical corticosteroids and severe disease (ulcers > 3 cm) that present with severe pain need to be treated with systemic medications such as corticosteroids or cyclosporine.
- Be careful when diagnosing peristomal pyoderma gangrenosum as this is overdiagnosed when it is just due to excessive granulation tissue.
- This is a neutrophilic dermatosis.

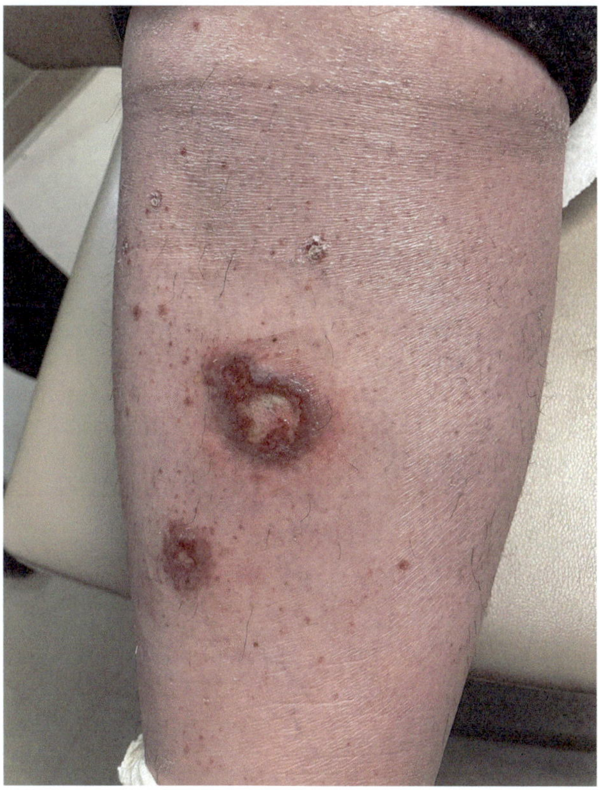

80. Pyogenic granuloma

- Morphology/clinical features
  - Solitary bright red, friable papule or polyp that easily bleeds.
    - Sometimes with epidermal collarette.
- Distribution
  - Most common sites (in decreasing order of frequency) are the gingiva, fingers, lips, face, and tongue.
    - Can also be seen on the trunk and extremities.
- Etiology/pathogenesis
  - A benign vascular neoplasm that likely arises from reactive neovascularization.
- Internal sequelae/comorbidities
  - a/w pregnancy.
- Laboratory testing
  - None.
- Treatments/prognosis
  - Shave excision under local anesthesia with electrodessication of the base of the lesion.
- USMLE Board Review Pearls
  - Look for the characteristic morphology on the fingers, trunk, or oral mucosa of a young adult.
  - Also known as a lobulated/lobular capillary hemangioma.
  - Lesions commonly ulcerate and bleed even with minor trauma.
  - Seen in pregnancy.
    - This is likely due to an increase in VEGF.
    - Lesions that form in pregnancy may self-resolve.
    - The most common site in a pregnant woman is on the oral mucosa or gingiva.
  - If a patient refuses shave excision, the lesion can be treated with silver nitrate, which will acutely reduce bleeding episodes and may shrink the lesion.
  - OCPs may increase the risk of forming these lesions.

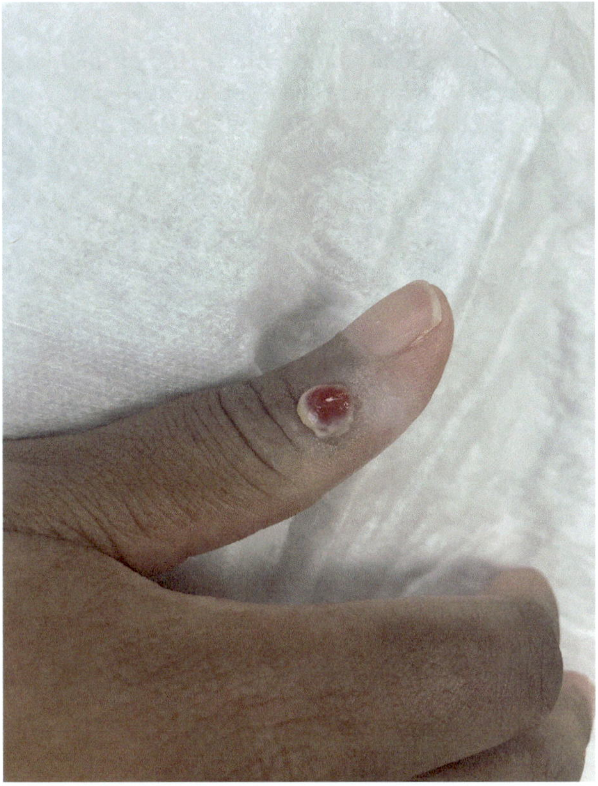

81. Rosacea

- Morphology/clinical features/distribution
  - There are several subtypes and variants of rosacea.
    - The four major subtypes will be covered here.
  - Erythematotelangiectatic = fixed erythema and telangiectasias on the face. Patients may complain of transient flushing.
  - Papulopustular = papules and pustules on an erythematous patch, lacking comedones, on the face.
  - Phymatous = thickened and pronounced skin most commonly seen on the nose (rhinophyma) but can involve the chin, forehead, earlobes, and eyelids.
  - Ocular = dryness, foreign body sensation, "gritty" sensation, burning/stinging sensation in the eyes.

- Etiology/pathogenesis
  - Inflammatory condition of the facial skin with multifactorial etiology, including vascular hyperreactivity, sensitivity to heat, hyperirritable/sensitive skin, and possible association with *Demodex* mites.
- Internal sequelae/comorbidities
  - None.
- Laboratory testing
  - None.
- Treatments/prognosis
  - Photoprotection and avoidance of triggers (patients usually report the following as common triggers: sunlight, heat/cold, stress, strong emotions, alcohol, hot beverages, and spicy foods).
  - Topical and oral antibiotics, topical metronidazole, and topical sodium sulfacetamide for the papulopustular subtype.
  - PDL laser and topical brimonidine for erythematotelangiectatic subtype.
- USMLE Board Review Pearls
  - Look for erythema, telangiectasias, and papules/pustules on the face lacking comedones. The characteristic patient is a middle-aged female with fair skin who presents to the dermatologist with "adult-onset acne."
  - Any rosacea patient may have ocular involvement that needs to be elicited by history. These patients require systemic therapy with PO doxycycline.
  - Alcohol and heat are some of the most common triggers for worsening rosacea.
  - Ocular rosacea may lead to chalazion/stye formation and blepharitis.
  - Know the four main subtypes of rosacea!
  - Laser therapy (CO_2 laser) is a treatment option for rhinophyma.

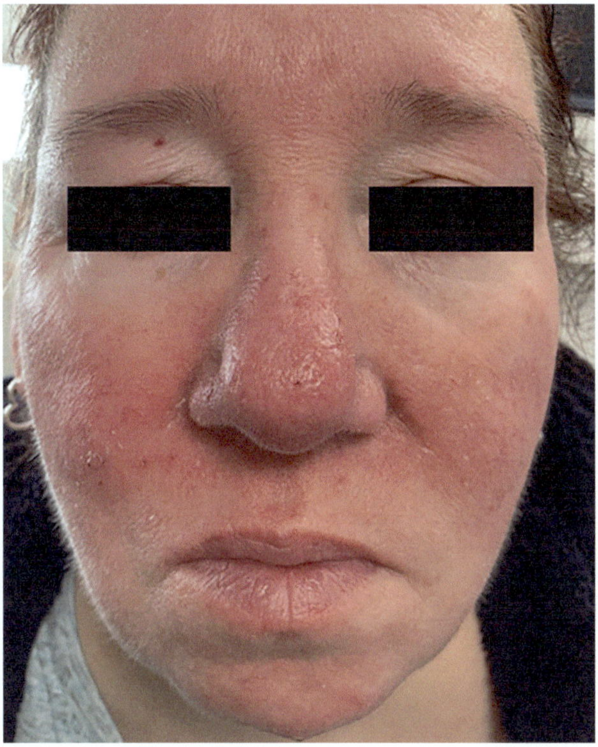

82. Sarcoidosis

- Morphology/clinical features
  - Classically presents as red-brown, nonscaly papules and plaques with a "dermal" feel.
  - Sarcoidosis is one of the great mimickers in dermatology!
    - Other less common and varied presentations include hypopigmented, ichthyosiform, angiolupoid, psoriasiform, annular, verrucous, cicatricial alopecia, and erythrodermic.
  - Lupus pernio is an important variant of sarcoidosis that presents with violaceous/red-brown beaded papules and plaques with a predilection for the nose, ears lobes, and cheeks.
    - Do not confuse Lupus pernio (sarcoid variant) with Lupus miliaris disseminatus faciei (rosacea variant) with Lupus vulgaris (tuberculosis) with Lupus erythematosus (autoimmune disease)!
    - This subtype is associated with more severe sarcoidosis of the lungs, sarcoidosis involving the upper respiratory tract and edema of the phalanges.

- Distribution
  - Predilection for the face and upper half of the body.
  - Sarcoidosis loves to form in preexisting scars, piercings, or tattoos.
- Etiology/pathogenesis
  - Multisystem granulomatous disease primarily driven by an upregulation of CD4+ Th1 cells to an unknown antigen.
- Internal sequelae/comorbidities
  - 90% of patients have lung involvement manifested by alveolitis, bronchiolitis, and pleuritis, which may result in "honeycombing" of lung, leading to fibrosis and bronchiectasis.
    - Ask any patient with suspected cutaneous sarcoidosis, "Do you have any lung problems?" and consider ordering a chest X-ray.
    - Look for hilar or paratracheal lymphadenopathy as well.
  - Up to half of sarcoidosis patients will have eye involvement manifested by anterior uveitis (most common) and inflammation of the eye, which may lead to blindness.
- Laboratory testing
  - ACE level (more useful in monitoring response to treatment than for diagnosis).
  - ESR; hypercalcemia and lymphopenia (increased).
- Treatments/prognosis
  - Difficult to treat and cure!
    - Cutaneous sarcoidosis = "you will die with this disease, not of this disease."
    - You do not need to treat cutaneous sarcoidosis unless it is disfiguring (i.e., involving the face) or painful (i.e., ulcerative).
    - In many cases, the treatment for cutaneous sarcoidosis is worse than the disease.
  - First line is PO corticosteroids for systemic involvement co-managed with the patient's primary care physician.
    - This will treat the cutaneous disease, but it will flare up again.
  - For skin predominant disease can try ILK, hydroxychloroquine, TNF-α inhibitors, and leflunomide, but there is limited efficacy.
- USMLE Board Review Pearls
  - On the exam, a patient with sarcoidosis will present with all or some of the following physical exam findings with or without skin involvement:

dyspnea, bilateral hilar lymphadenopathy on chest imaging, noncaseating granulomas on pathology, increased ACE levels, and hypercalcemia.

- Hypercalcemia can be explained by the following mechanism: noncaseating granulomas lead to macrophage activity, which causes increased 1α-hydroxylase activity in macrophages, leading to vitamin D activation and causing an increase in calcium.

– Sarcoidosis is a/w erythema nodosum, and this is a positive prognostic factor for the disease.
– Systemic sarcoidosis can impact the heart.
– Every patient who is diagnosed with cutaneous sarcoidosis should have their lungs and eyes examined and a have a full physical exam and laboratory evaluation by their primary care doctor.
– Lupus pernio is strongly associated with chronic sarcoidosis of the lung and upper respiratory tract disease.

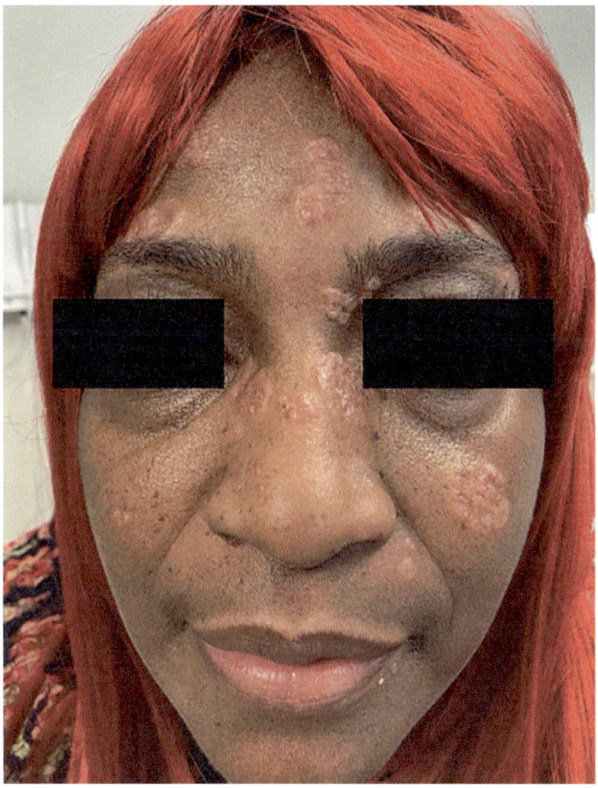

83. Scabies

- Morphology/clinical features
  - Small erythematous papules, excoriations, and "burrows," which are described as wavy, thread-like, grayish-white linear plaques that are a few millimeters in length.
  - Patient will complain of severe and eruptive pruritus that is worse at night and with hot showers.
  - Crusted scabies presents as thick plaques with "sandpaper"-like scale that is sometimes misdiagnosed as psoriasis due to the prominent/thick scale.
  - Penile nodular scabies presents as erythematous papules and nodules on the penis and scrotum.
- Distribution
  - Classically involves the interdigital web spaces of the hands, flexural aspect of the wrists, axillae, posterior auricular area, waist (including the umbilicus), ankles, feet, and buttocks.
- Etiology/pathogenesis
  - Caused by *sarcoptes scabiei var. hominis* mite.
- Internal sequelae/comorbidities
  - Secondary bacterial infections.
- Laboratory testing
  - Skin scraping with mineral oil preparation and evaluation with a light microscope.
- Treatments/prognosis
  - Easily treatable with topical or oral medications. Patients may require multiple rounds of treatment for successful eradication and pruritus may take up to 2–4 weeks or months to resolve (post-scabetic itch) but improvement may be noticed in days.
    - Common medications include permethrin cream, spinosad suspension, and PO ivermectin.
  - Counsel patient on infectious nature of the condition and to wash all clothing and bedding in hot water.
  - In confirmed cases of scabies, family members and close contacts should be treated, even if they are asymptomatic, as the incubation period may last up to 6 weeks.
- USMLE Board Review Pearls
  - Look for pinpoint erythematous papules and linear to curvy erythematous lines in the characteristic areas, especially the webspace of the fingers and

toes. Patients will complain of intense pruritus, and sometimes all that is seen is excoriations on the skin.

- Scabies is transmitted by close skin-to-skin contact and is more commonly found in overcrowded populations such as nursing homes, prisons, and homeless shelters.
- Must address the clothing/bedding as well as the patient.
- Crusted scabies is more commonly seen in immunocompromised patients (i.e., HIV patients).
- 5% permethrin cream should be applied neck down over the entire body, washed off in the morning, and repeated in 1 week. This treatment is usually combined with PO ivermectin.
- Scabies mites cannot be seen with naked eye as opposed to lice.
- Secondary bacterial infections are common due to scratching.
- Permethrin cream may cause an allergic contact dermatitis in patients who have a sensitivity to formaldehyde or who are allergic to chrysanthemums. This is rarely seen in clinical practice.

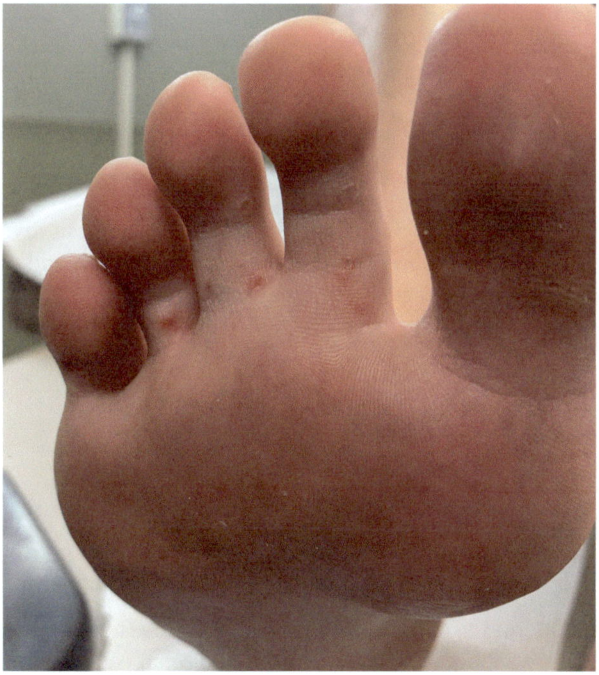

84. Scleroderma (systemic sclerosis)

- Morphology/clinical features
  - Basic feature that is common to both limited and diffuse scleroderma is "stiff" or "tight" skin.
  - Initial presenting sign is skin thickening and edema of the digits, leading to taut and shiny skin on the fingers.
    - Can lead to flexion contractures.
    - Digital tip ulcers.
  - Telangiectasias
    - Classically described as "matted" (squared off) and more common in limited scleroderma.
  - Hypopigmented patches with perifollicular hyperpigmentation ("salt and pepper skin").
- Distribution
  - Limited = "limited" to distal extremities and face.
  - Diffuse = "diffusely" involving distal/proximal extremities, face, and trunk.
  - "Salt and pepper skin" most commonly seen on the upper trunk and face.
- Etiology/pathogenesis
  - Multifactorial pathophysiology including vascular dysfunction and immune dysregulation leading to excessive collagen and protein production/deposition in skin and internal organs.
- Internal sequelae/comorbidities
  - Limited
    - a/w pulmonary artery hypertension.
  - Diffuse
    - a/w interstitial lung disease (ILD).
      - **Diffuse** scleroderma **diffusely** impacts the lungs.
  - Other internal comorbidities include cardiovascular (myocardial fibrosis), GI (dysphagia and dysmotility), and renal (scleroderma renal crisis).
- Laboratory testing
  - Limited = (+) anti-centromere antibody.
  - Diffuse = (+) anti-SCL-70 antibody.

- Treatments/prognosis
  - 10-year survival is 70% for limited and 50% for diffuse.
  - There is no highly effective treatment for the cutaneous manifestations of scleroderma. These patients should be referred to rheumatology/internal medicine to manage the internal comorbidities.
    - The most important role of the dermatologist is to make the diagnosis and refer to the appropriate specialists.
  - ILD is the number 1 cause of death due to control of scleroderma renal crisis with ACEi.
- USMLE Board Review Pearls
  - Look for symmetric, thickened, puffy, taut skin of the face and distal extremities.
    - Limited form will be limited to the head, neck, and distal extremities.
    - Diffuse form will involve the chest, abdomen, and extremities.
  - **C**REST syndrome is a variant of limited scleroderma, and anti-**C**entromere antibodies are indicative of this syndrome.
    - CREST syndrome is characterized by **C**alcinosis cutis, **R**aynaud phenomenon, **E**sophageal dysmotility, **S**clerodactyly, and **T**elangiectasias.
  - Important internal manifestations of diffuse scleroderma include GI dysmotility, pulmonary fibrosis, and renal failure.
  - Scleroderma renal crisis is seen as an acute onset of renal failure and hypertension in a scleroderma patient.
    - Must recognize this and treat promptly as there is a high mortality rate!
    - Treat with ACEi.
  - > 90% of patients with scleroderma will have a positive ANA.
  - Anti-Scl-70/anti-topoisomerase-I is highly specific but not sensitive to diffuse scleroderma.
  - Mortality is most commonly due to pulmonary or renal complications.
  - RNA polymerase III autoantibodies in scleroderma indicate renal involvement.
  - Treatment of scleroderma should be co-managed with rheumatology/internal medicine as there are few therapies that can effectively treat the cutaneous manifestations of this disease.

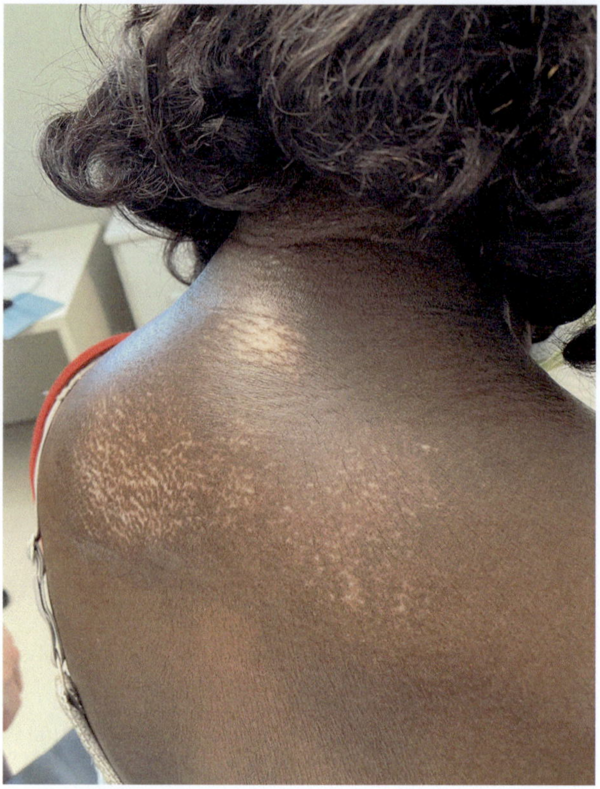

85. Seborrheic dermatitis

- Morphology/clinical features
  - Well-defined salmon-colored/red plaques with yellow, greasy scale.
  - Petaloid seborrheic dermatitis is a variant that presents with well-defined round/oval, polycyclic, and arcuate plaques on the head and neck area.
  - Dandruff is a mild form of seborrheic dermatitis characterized by flaking and itching of the scalp.
- Distribution
  - Favors highly sebaceous areas including scalp, eyebrows, nasolabial folds, ears/retroauricular area, and central chest.
- Etiology/pathogenesis
  - Inflammation due to the overgrowth of *Malassezia*.

- Internal sequelae/comorbidities
  - In severe cases, check for HIV or Parkinson's disease.
- Laboratory testing
  - None.
- Treatments/prognosis
  - Topical corticosteroids, topical azoles, ketoconazole shampoo, and topical selenium sulfide.
  - 0.3% roflumilast topical foam is FDA approved for seborrheic dermatitis.
- USMLE Board Review Pearls
  - Look for well-defined erythematous plaques with yellowish, large, greasy scale involving the eyebrows, scalp, and nasolabial folds.
  - Seb derm is thought to partially occur due to an inflammatory reaction to *Malassezia,* which is part of normal skin flora.
  - Be careful diagnosing seb derm in a pre-pubertal patient! Must rule out tinea capitis first.
  - Seb derm commonly presents in infants and is known as "cradle cap" on the scalp. It can also affect the diaper area and should be included in the differential for "diaper rash."
    - Treat cradle cap with frequent shampooing, baby or mineral oil and frequent brushing/combing.
  - Extensive seb derm is a/w HIV, Parkinson's disease, and mood disorders (depression, psychosis).
  - The medical term for dandruff is pityriasis simplex capillitii.
    - Treat with topical steroid solution and ketoconazole shampoo.
    - The ketoconazole shampoo may leave the hair very dry, recommend to use a conditioner afterward.
    - The more the patient washes their hair, the more effective the ketoconazole shampoo will be.

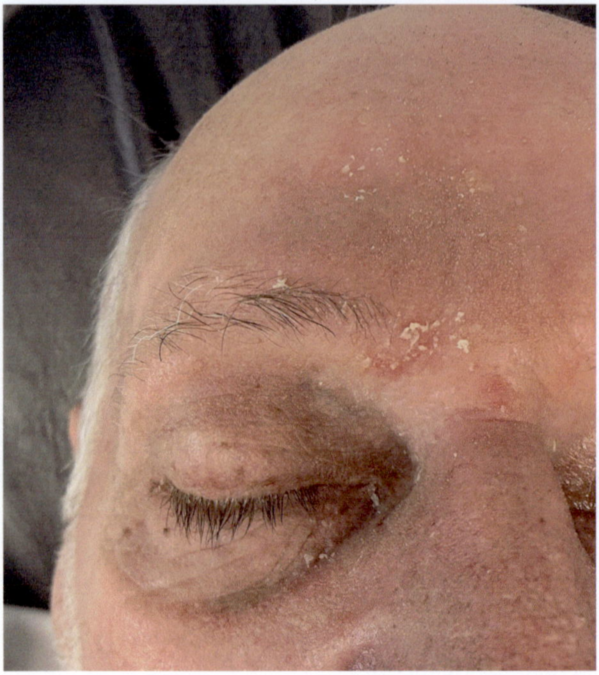

86. Seborrheic keratosis (SK)

- Morphology/clinical features
  - Well-demarcated dark brown/black waxy, verrucous/pebbly papule, or plaque with a "stuck-on" appearance.
  - Dermatosis papulosis nigra is an SK variant in darker skin patients characterized by numerous, small SK-like lesions on the face/neck.
    - Look at a picture of the actor Morgan Freeman.
- Distribution
  - Face, trunk, and extremities.
  - Spares mucosal sites.
- Etiology/pathogenesis
  - Associated with sun exposure and aging.
  - Mutations in *FGFR3* and *PIK3CA*.
- Internal sequelae/comorbidities
  - Sign of Leser-Trélat = widespread eruption of SKs on the trunk due to underlying adenocarcinoma.
    - In everyday clinical practice, this phenomenon is very rare.

- Laboratory testing
  - None.
- Treatments/prognosis
  - Shave excision or cryotherapy.
- USMLE Board Review Pearls
  - Look for a well-demarcated brown/black, pebbly papule on the skin of a patient 50 years old or older.
  - The number 1 underlying adenocarcinoma in the sign of Leser-Trélat is GI adenocarcinoma.
  - There is 0% risk that an SK will develop into cancer but patients are often referred to the dermatologist for malignancy concern.
  - Irritated SKs have a rim of erythema around them from minor trauma or excoriations.

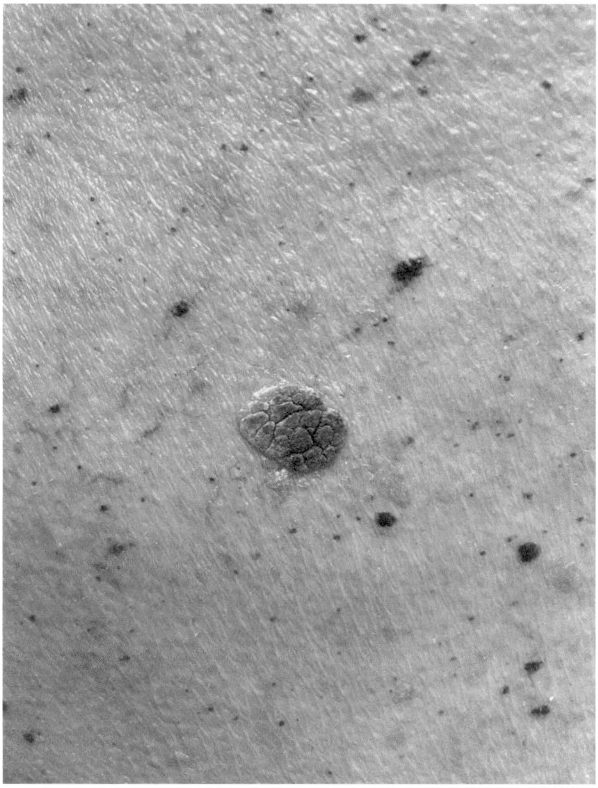

87. Staph scaled skin syndrome (SSSS)

- Morphology/clinical features/distribution
  - Begins on the face (periorificial erythema and fissuring) and intertriginous zone with a febrile prodrome.
    - These patients have a look of an “unhappy clown” due to the redness, scaling and edema around the eyes and corners of the mouth.
    - They will be frowning due to skin tenderness, fever, and malaise.
  - Progresses to widespread erythematous and wrinkled appearing skin with easily ruptured flaccid bullae.
  - Results in desquamation and heals without scarring.
- Etiology/pathogenesis
  - *S. aureus* produces exfoliatoxins A & B, which leads to cleavage of desmoglein 1, causing a subcorneal split in the skin.
- Internal sequelae/comorbidities
  - Seen in adults with chronic renal failure.
- Laboratory testing
  - The skin is sterile.
    - Culture the nasopharynx or conjunctivae (most common site of primary infection).
- Treatments/prognosis
  - Good prognosis.
  - Treat with dicloxacillin or cephalexin.
  - Severe cases require hospitalization and IV antibiotics.
- USMLE Board Review Pearls
  - Look for the “unhappy clown” face in a young patient.
  - This disease is most common in infants and young children.
    - Do not diagnose an adult with SSSS unless they have chronic renal failure!
  - SSSS can be thought of as “generalized bullous impetigo” because the same exfoliatoxins cause both diseases but in SSSS these toxins are hematogenously disseminated.
  - Do not culture the skin, it will be negative. Culture the nasopharynx because that is likely where the source of the *staph* bacteria is.
  - There is no mucosal involvement but there is a positive Nikolsky sign.
  - At the histological level, there is acantholysis in the granular layer of the epidermis.

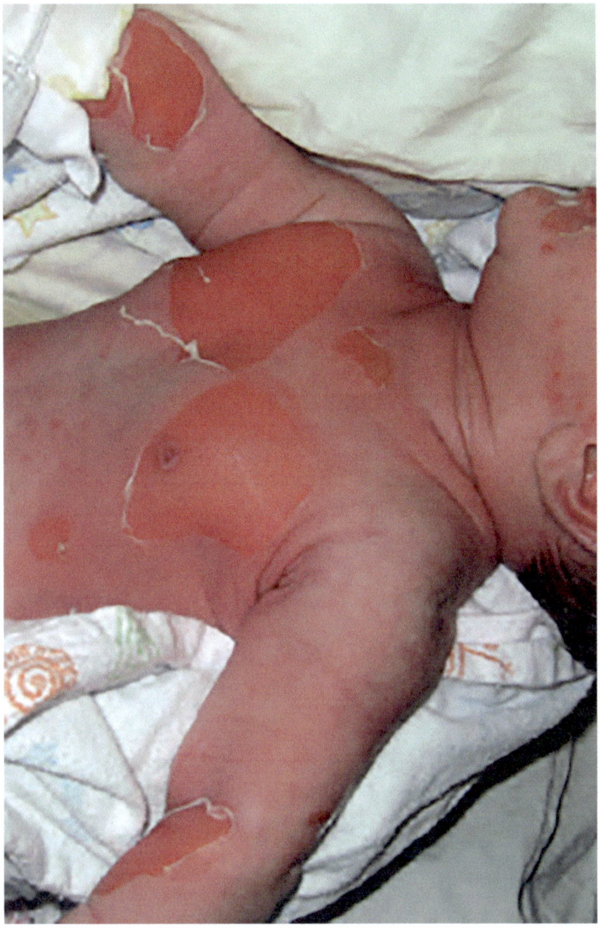

88. Stasis dermatitis/lipodermatosclerosis (LDS)

- Morphology/clinical features
  - Stasis dermatitis—scaling, erythema, edema, dyspigmentation (hemosiderin pigmentation), and inflammation.
  - LDS—end-stage stasis dermatitis involving the skin and subcutaneous tissue manifested by very firm, indurated plaques with intense hemosiderin pigmentation and changes of atrophie blanche giving the appearance of an "inverted wine bottle" on the leg (you can use the term "inverted champagne bottle" if you are feeling particularly fancy).
  - Acroangiodermatitis of Mali ("pseudo-Kaposi sarcoma") is a rare type of stasis dermatitis seen on the lower extremities that may mimic Kaposi sarcoma because it is violaceus/purple in color.

- Distribution
  - Lower extremities.
- Etiology/pathogenesis
  - Chronic venous hypertension from valvular incompetence of deep leg veins leading to capillary barrier permeability and leakage of fluid and plasma proteins into the surrounding tissue.
    - Look for varicosities, including venulectasias of the instep as a cutaneous sign of chronic venous hypertension.
- Internal sequelae/comorbidities
  - Venous stasis ulcers are very difficult to heal and require extensive wound care.
    - A venous stasis ulcer has irregular borders with a shallow, yellow fibrinous base classically above the medial malleolus.
- Laboratory testing
  - None.
- Treatments/prognosis
  - For the dermatitis, can use topical corticosteroids.
  - Need to address the underlying venous stasis with compression stockings, leg elevation, and referral to vascular surgery.
  - Try to avoid performing a skin biopsy on LDS, a large percentage of wounds will not heal well.
- USMLE Board Review Pearls
  - Venous stasis ulcers typically occur in the "gaiter area," which is the ankle to mid-calf typically over the malleoli, have shallow/irregular borders, and are associated with venous stasis changes in the background.
  - Arterial ulcers have a symmetric/circular, well-defined punched-out appearance at pressure points and distal toes (where circulation is poor). The surrounding skin will be pale, cold, and atrophic as a result of poor circulation.
  - Secondary to venous hypertension from venous valve incompetence or flow obstruction. Patients usually have a history of standing for long periods of time.
  - Treat by addressing the underlying cause (leg elevation, compression stockings) and topical steroids for pruritus and inflammation.
  - Hyperpigmentation in this condition is due to hemosiderin deposition.
  - Another name for LDS is sclerosing panniculitis and essentially there is fat necrosis from severe venous stasis.

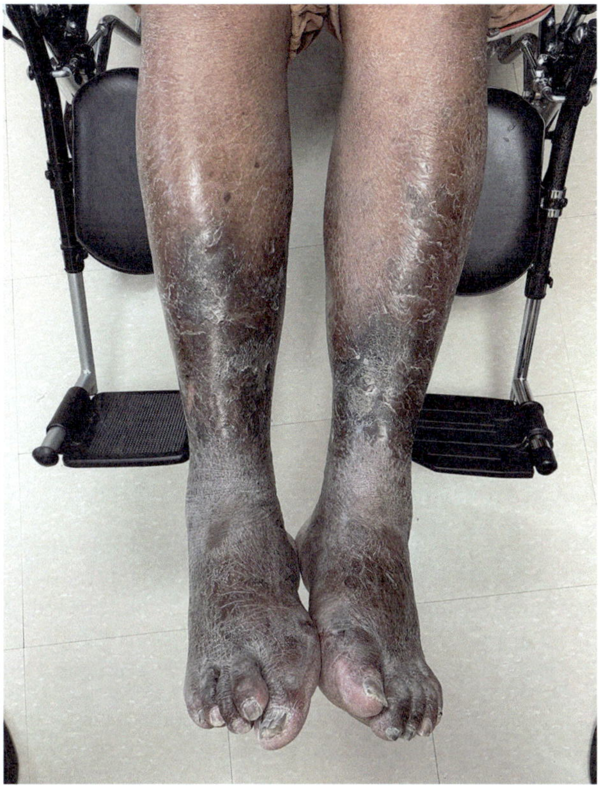

89. Sunburn/photoaging

- Morphology/clinical features/distribution
  - Sunburn = erythema and peeling and occasionally bullae formation on sun-exposed areas of the skin, including the face, trunk, and upper extremities.
  - Solar elastosis = thickened, wrinkled, yellowish skin on sun-exposed areas.
  - Solar elastotic nodules/bands = yellowish nodules or plaques due to sun damage.
  - Cutis rhomboidalis nuchae = a form of solar elastosis involving the posterior neck with geometrically patterned leather-like, thick, wrinkled skin.
  - Poikiloderma of Civatte = reticular, patterned reddish-brown telangiectatic patches on the lateral neck (relatively sun-protected submental region is spared).
  - Favre–Racouchot syndrome = clusters of large open comedones on the lateral/inferior periorbital area/temple overlying skin with solar elastosis.
  - Colloid milium = 1–2 mm white-yellow subcutaneous papules (resembling milia), often grouped, on sun-exposed areas like the face and hands.

- Weathering nodules = 1–2 mm white-yellow subcutaneous, painless papules on the helix of the ears.
- Solar lentigines = multiple light to dark brown irregularly shaped macules on sun-exposed skin.

- Etiology/pathogenesis
  - Acute and chronic UV radiation exposure.
- Internal sequelae/comorbidities
  - Skin cancer and photoaging.
- Laboratory testing
  - None.
- Treatments/prognosis
  - Photoprotection with sun avoidance and sunscreen.
    - Patients should be counseled to use a broad-spectrum sunscreen with a sun protection factor (SPF) of at least 30 applied a half hour prior to exposure. Reapplication of sunscreen should occur every 2 hours, especially after swimming or sweating. Ideally, the amount of sunscreen used at each application should fill a standard shot glass.
      - If a patient says their bottle of sunscreen lasts them the entire summer, they are not using it properly!
- USMLE Board Review Pearls
  - A sunburn is a first-degree burn of the skin and is an acute cutaneous inflammatory reaction due to excessive UV irradiation.
  - UVB predominantly contributes to sunburn and UVA predominantly contributes to photoaging.
    - **B** for **B**urning and **A** for **A**ging.
  - Treat mild sunburn with cool, moist compresses, and emollients with aloe vera for topical relief. Can also use NSAIDs for pain relief.
  - It is important to recognize the many forms of photoaging discussed above to avoid unnecessary workup.
  - Know how to properly counsel a patient on best practices for photoprotection/sunscreen use.

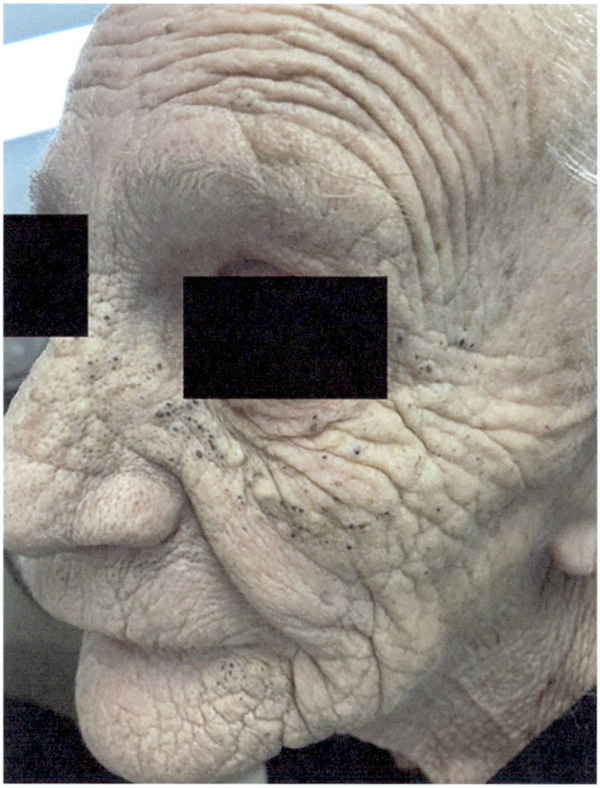

90. Sweet syndrome (acute febrile neutrophilic dermatosis)

- Morphology/clinical features
  - Erythematous, edematous, "juicy" papules and plaques a/w tenderness and burning pain.
  - Patients will likely present with a fever, leukocytosis, and arthralgias/arthritis.
- Distribution
  - Favors the head/neck and upper extremities.
  - Wrong distribution is not a dealbreaker; cases have been described involving other areas of the body as well.
- Etiology/pathogenesis
  - Unknown but the pathophysiology is thought to involve a hypersensitivity reaction.
  - Various triggers

    - Infections (*strep* and yersinosis)
    - Cancer (AML, other hematologic and solid malignancies)
    - IBD
    - Drugs (G-CSF, GM-CSF, ATRA, Bactrim, OCPs)
        - Rare cause
    - Other (autoimmune diseases)

- Internal sequelae/comorbidities
    - a/w IBD, URI infection, malignancies (most common is AML), and polycythemia vera.
- Laboratory testing
    - CBC, ESR/CRP
- Treatments/prognosis
    - Treatment of choice is systemic steroids.
    - Resolves without scarring but can recur.
- USMLE Board Review Pearls
    - Look for erythematous, edematous plaques on the arms and neck of a middle-aged female with a history of cancer or infection. The patient will complain of burning pain.
    - Sweet syndrome is a neutrophilic dermatosis and on histopathology there is a robust neutrophilic infiltrate.
    - First-line therapy and treatment of choice is systemic steroids.
        - Systemic steroids should lead to rapid relief.
    - Must determine the underlying cause, and, in many cases, patients will require a malignancy work-up.
    - The most common ocular finding in Sweet syndrome is conjunctivitis.

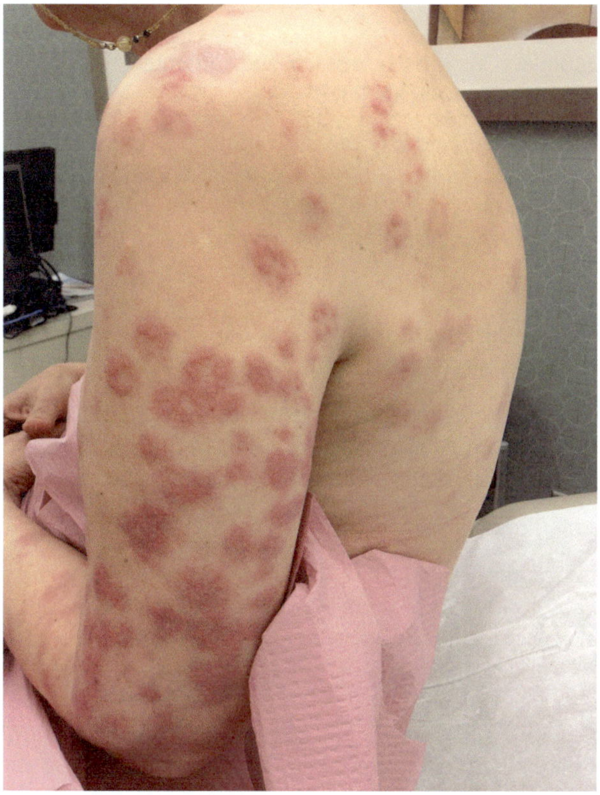

91. Syphilis

- Morphology/clinical features/distribution
  - Primary—**painless**, well-demarcated ulcer on the genitals (chancre).
  - Secondary—acute, papulosquamous eruption of round "copper-colored" scaly, macules and papules on the trunk, extremities, and acral surfaces.
    - Erupts 3–10 weeks after untreated primary syphilis.
    - Lesion size is referred to as "nickel and dime."
    - The scale of secondary syphilis is classically described as thick, peripheral, and off-white.
      - This is called "biette" scale of syphilis.
    - Other secondary presentations include "moth-eaten" alopecia of the scalp and condyloma lata (smooth, moist plaques in the genital region).
    - Syphilis is nonvesicular in an adult patient.
- Etiology/pathogenesis
  - Caused by *Treponema pallidum,* a gram-negative spirochete.

- Internal sequelae/comorbidities
  - If secondary syphilis is missed and untreated, it could lead to tertiary syphilis months to years later.
    - This is manifested by the involvement of the nervous system (neurosyphilis), cardiovascular system (aortitis), and musculoskeletal system (gummas).
    - Argyll–Robertson pupil—accommodates to light but does not react.
- Laboratory testing
  - Serologic studies are divided into treponemal (FTA-ABS, TPPA) and non-treponemal (RPR,VDRL).
    - Most sensitive and specific tests are the treponemal tests.
    - Start with an RPR as a screening test as this is the first test to become positive and usually will become negative after successful treatment.
- Treatments/prognosis
  - IM benzathine PCN (2.4M IU x 1 dose) for primary and secondary disease and follow-up of titers (usually with an infectious disease referral).
  - An alternative choice for therapy is doxycycline 100 mg BID for 2 weeks.
  - IV PCN for tertiary syphilis.
- USMLE Board Review Pearls
  - Syphilis is extremely high yield on exams! It can be a congenital infection and can impact a patient at any age. Know how to diagnose syphilis clinically and understand how laboratory testing works along with its limitations and pitfalls.
  - Syphilis is one of the "great mimickers" in medicine and can have many various presentations both on the skin and systemically.
  - Look for a painless, indurated ulcer on the genitals of a sexually active patient or an acute eruption of round, scaly, "copper-colored lesions" on the trunk, extremities, palms, and soles of a sexually active patient.
    - This presentation may mimic pityriasis rosea.
  - Condyloma lata are smooth, moist, painless, wart-like lesion on the genitals of a patient with secondary syphilis.
    - Do not confuse with condyloma acuminatum, which is a genital wart caused by HPV virus.
  - Gummas are chronic granulomas of the skin and bones in tertiary syphilis.
  - Signs of tertiary neurosyphilis are broad-based ataxia, tabes dorsalis, "general paresis," Charcot joints, and positive Romberg's sign.
  - False-positive non-treponemal syphilis test can be seen with the following conditions: pregnancy, viral infections (EBV), SLE, and leprosy.

- Direct testing includes darkfield microscopy and PCR.
- Indirect testing includes non-treponemal tests (RPR, VDRL) and treponemal tests (FTA-ABS, TPPA).
  - Non-treponemal test titers revert to zero after successful treatment.
  - Treponemal tests will remain positive.
- Syphilis is a reportable disease to the local health department.
  - Other reportable sexually transmitted infections are gonorrhea, chlamydia, chancroid, and HIV.

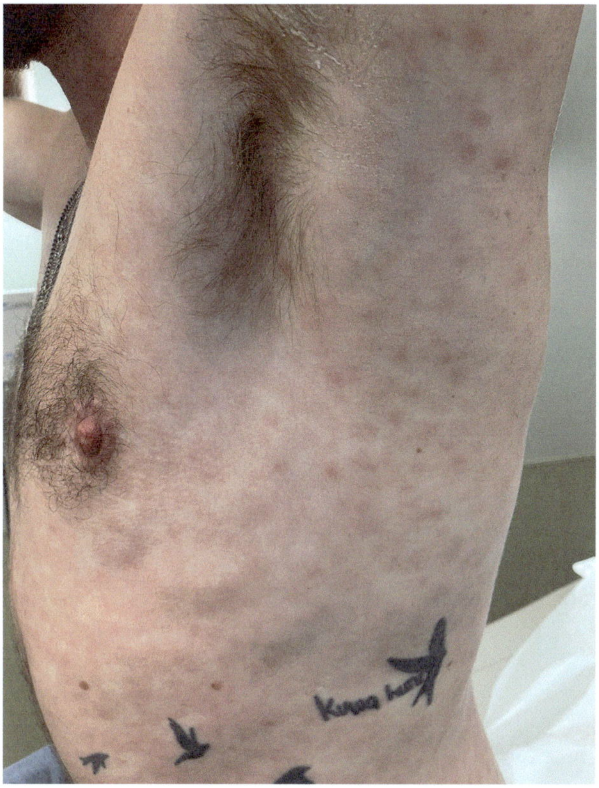

92. Syringoma

- Morphology/clinical features
  - Multiple skin-colored to translucent, yellow-tinged papules.
- Distribution
  - Periorbital region and sometimes cheeks.
    - Can occur anywhere but these sites are most common.
- Etiology/pathogenesis
  - Benign adnexal neoplasm that is of eccrine origin.
- Internal sequelae/comorbidities
  - Clear cell syringomas are a/w diabetes.
- Laboratory testing
  - None.
- Treatments/prognosis
  - Cryosurgery, punch excision, or electrosurgical destruction.
- USMLE Board Review Pearls
  - Look for multiple, similar appearing small skin-colored papules around the eyes bilaterally.
  - There is an increased incidence in females, Asian patients, and Down syndrome patients.
  - The eyelids are the number 1 most common site.
  - Clear cell syringoma (which is a histological diagnosis and not a clinical diagnosis) is a/w diabetes.

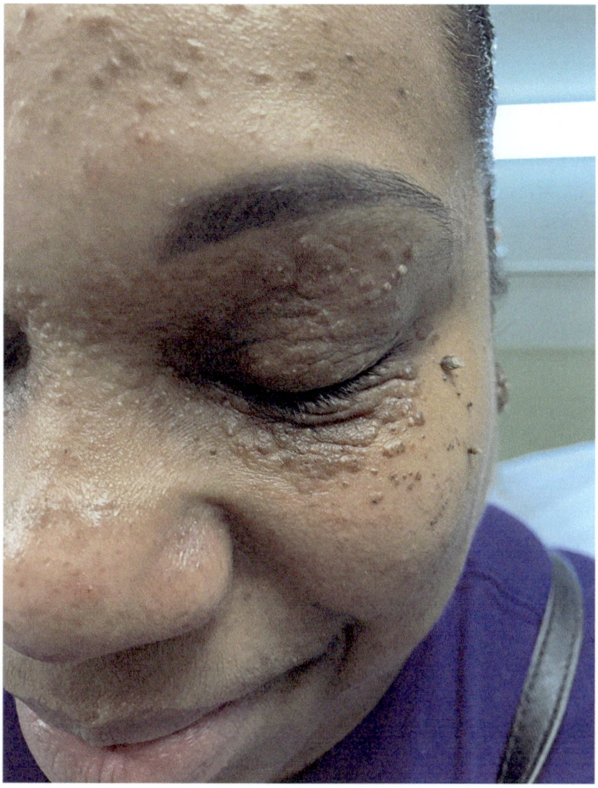

93. Telogen effluvium

- Morphology/clinical features
  - Patients will complain of hair shedding without obvious or discrete areas of hair loss.
- Distribution
  - Scalp.
- Etiology/pathogenesis
  - A triggering event by an unknown mechanism causes the hair to enter the telogen phase and ~3 months later the exogen phase when the hair begins to shed.
    - Triggers include the following: thyroid disease, iron deficiency, pregnancy/postpartum, severe stressful event (death in family, divorce), surgery, high fever, illness, COVID-19, and malnutrition.
    - Medications—OCPs, retinoids, anticonvulsants, heavy metals, and beta-blockers.

- Internal sequelae/comorbidities
  - None.
- Laboratory testing
  - In unexplained cases of hair loss when a trigger cannot be identified, hair loss experts recommend checking CBC, TSH, ferritin, metabolic panel, and ESR.
    - Serum ferritin levels should be corrected to at least 40 ng/dl, but the relationship of reduced iron stores and hair loss still has not been elucidated.
  - Hair pull test = 4-6 telogen hair are elicited after gently pulling on about 40 hairs.
- Treatments/prognosis
  - Counsel the patient that they will not go bald and this condition will self-resolve.
  - In some cases, chronic telogen effluvium can last years to decades.
  - Can try oral or topical minoxidil to encourage hair growth.
- USMLE Board Review Pearls
  - This condition classically presents in a patient who complains of excessive hair shedding after a triggering event 3 months earlier.
  - There will be no obvious or discrete areas of hair loss; the patient will look normal upon entering the exam room.
  - Other hair-bearing regions on the body may be affected as well.
  - Treatment of choice is counseling and supportive care with laboratory testing in cases when a trigger cannot be identified.
  - While there is some overlap in triggers, do not confuse telogen effluvium with anagen effluvium.
    - Anagen effluvium is most commonly seen with chemotherapy when there is abrupt and simultaneous inhibition of the mitotic activity of follicular matrix cells leading to acute and nearly complete hair loss (this is why chemotherapy patients go bald).
      - The anagen phase is arrested and the telogen phase is unaffected.

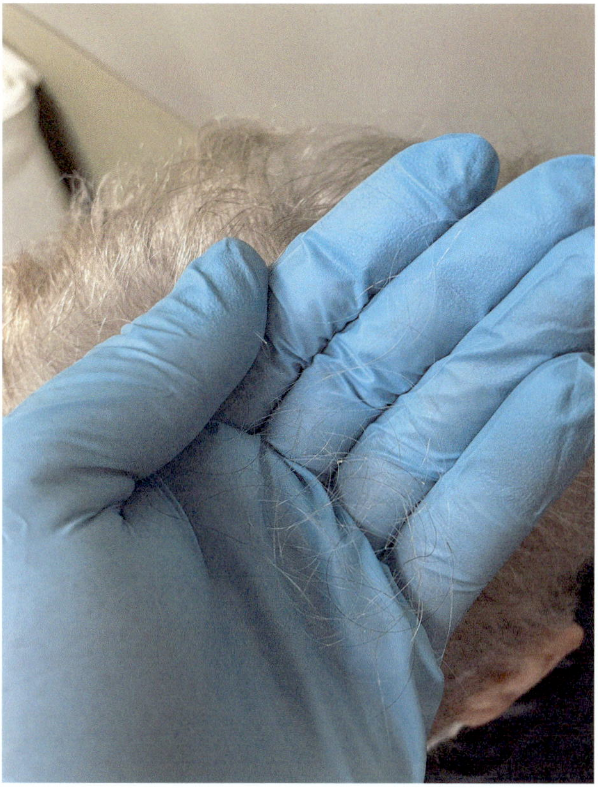

94. Tinea corporis (dermatophyte)
    - Morphology/clinical features
        - Annular or **serpiginous** scaly plaque with **active/inflamed border** and central clearing.
            - This is often confused with asteatotic eczema.
                - Asteatotic eczema has a more prominent cracked, dry look throughout the entire plaque, and the border will not be as active/inflamed as in tinea corporis.
                - Sometimes asking the patient about new cats or guinea pigs at home will help steer you toward a diagnosis of tinea corporis while asking a patient about showering habits will help steer you toward a diagnosis of asteatotic eczema (the patient will endorse taking daily to sometimes twice daily long > 30 min, hot showers).
                - The nails can also be examined for onychomycosis which can help steer your diagnosis toward tinea corporis.

- Distribution
  - Favors the trunk, extremities, and groin.
- Etiology/pathogenesis
  - Most commonly caused by the dermatophyte *T. rubrum.*
- Internal sequelae/comorbidities
  - None.
- Laboratory testing
  - Can perform KOH prep to look for hyphae.
    - Make sure you know what a clothing fiber looks like on KOH prep so as to not falsely diagnose tinea corporis.
    - Thin branching hyphae should be crossing multiple skin cells on KOH prep.
- Treatments/prognosis
  - PO terbinafine
    - A common treatment regimen is 250 mg daily for 1 month.
- USMLE Board Review Pearls
  - Look for a serpiginous, erythematous scaly plaque with an active/red/inflamed/prominent border and central clearing.
  - Tinea corporis is caused by a dermatophyte which is a microorganism that invades fully keratinized tissue such as stratum corneum, hair and nails.
    - Dermatophytes include *Microsporum, Trichophyton*, and *Epidermophyton* species.
  - Tinea corporis is also known as "ringworm" and is sometimes contracted from infected pets (cats, guinea pigs).
  - Tinea pedis (athlete's foot) is a dermatophyte infection of the feet characterized by a scaly plaque in a "moccasin distribution" or interdigital scaly plaques.
    - Involvement of one hand is typical, and this is referred to as "two feet-one hand syndrome."
  - Tinea cruris (jock itch) is a dermatophyte infection of the groin with a similar morphology to tinea corporis.
    - Tinea cruris spares the scrotum as opposed to a candida infection, which will commonly impact the scrotum.

- Onychomycosis or tinea unguium is a dermatophyte infection of nails manifested by nail thickening, crumbling, subungual/yellowish debris, and nail dystrophy.
- Tinea capitis is a fungal infection of the scalp commonly seen in pediatric patients manifested by scaly plaques in areas of hair loss with lymphadenopathy. Tinea capitis in an adult patient is rare.
  - A kerion is a variant of tinea capitis manifested by a large, crusted, scaly, boggy, inflamed plaque on the scalp.

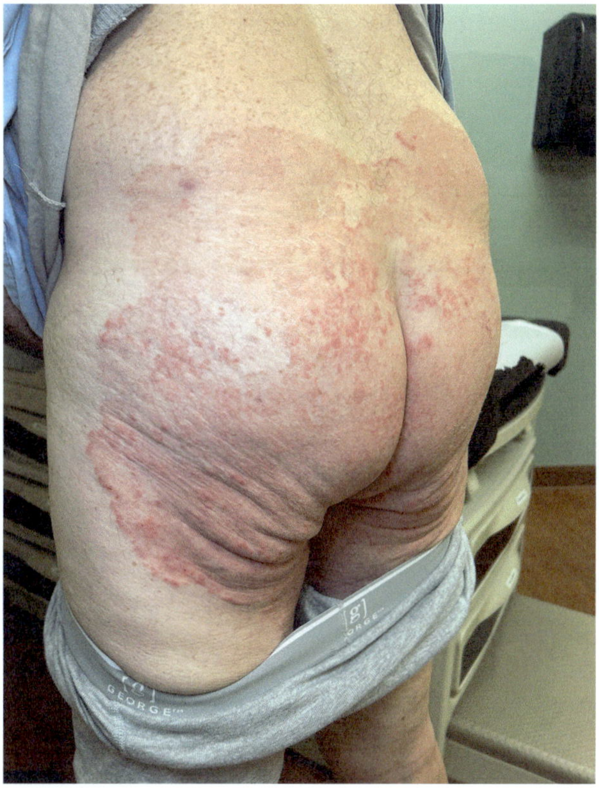

95. Tinea versicolor (pityriasis versicolor)
  - Morphology/clinical features
    - Hyperpigmented/light brown or hypopigmented finely scaling circular/oval macules/patches.
    - Sometimes they can be red in color.

- Distribution
  - Favors seborrheic areas and sun-exposed skin of the face, neck, upper trunk, and extremities.
- Etiology/pathogenesis
  - Caused by *Malassezia globosa* and *M. furfur*
    - Yeast form is normal skin flora; transforms to filamentous/hyphal form in the pathogenic state.
- Internal sequelae/comorbidities
  - None.
- Laboratory testing
  - KOH prep to look for "ziti and meatballs" (hyphae and spores).
- Treatments/prognosis
  - PO fluconazole, topical ketoconazole, and topical selenium sulfide.
- USMLE Board Review Pearls
  - Look for numerous light brown, finely scaling macules and patches on the trunk and extremities.
  - Caused by *Malassezia* and worsened by humid and sweaty conditions.
    - Tinea versicolor is a misnomer because *Malassezia* is a yeast and not a dermatophyte, which is why I prefer the more correct term of pityriasis versicolor.
  - Often more pronounced after sun exposure because these lesions fail to tan like normal skin due to the modulation of melanin production by the organism.

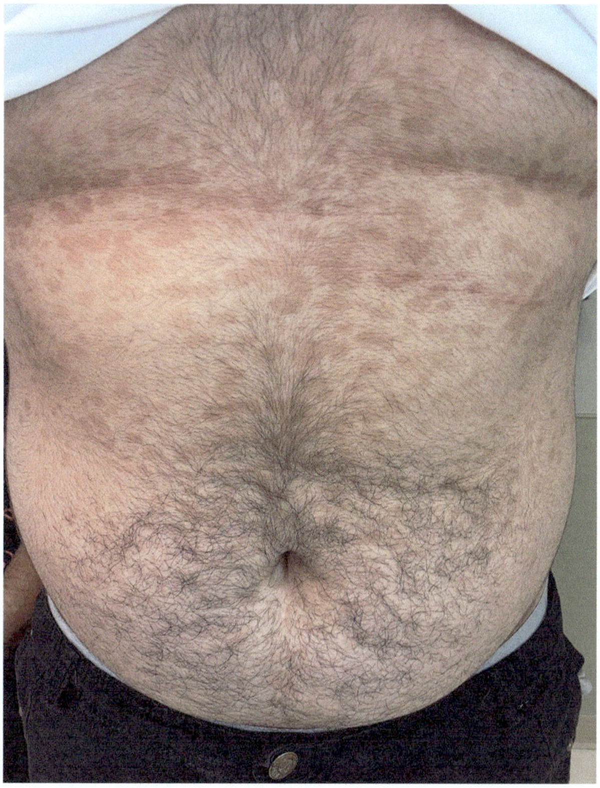

96. Urticaria

- Morphology/clinical features
  - Erythematous, pruritic, edematous papules, and plaques without surface change commonly referred to as a “wheal” or “hives.”
  - Individual lesions disappear within 24 hours.
    - Lesions are “here today and gone tomorrow.”
    - This is a hallmark of the disease but larger coalescing lesions may take longer to resolve.
  - Classified into acute urticaria and chronic urticaria.
    - Chronic urticaria is defined as twice weekly episodes greater than 6 weeks duration of treatment.
- Distribution
  - Commonly seen on the trunk, extremities, and face.

- Etiology/pathogenesis
  - Mast cell is the primary cell that is implicated in urticaria due to release of histamine through a degranulation stimulus.
  - Acute urticaria—50% of cases are idiopathic, 40% are due to URIs, 9% are due to medications, and 1% is due to foods.
  - Chronic urticaria—45% of cases are idiopathic, 25% are inducible urticarias (i.e., pressure, heat, cold, dermatographism), 20% are autoimmune in nature (patients have functional autoantibodies against FcεRI or the Fc portion of IgE), and 5% are infection related.
- Internal sequelae/comorbidities
  - a/w with autoimmune thyroid disease and other autoimmune conditions, such as vitiligo, diabetes, rheumatoid arthritis, and pernicious anemia.
  - Increased risk of hematologic malignancy, especially non-Hodgkin lymphoma, was noted in one large retrospective cohort study.
- Laboratory testing
  - None for routine cases.
  - For recalcitrant cases of chronic urticaria with no known causes consider CBC w/ differential, ESR/CRP, thyroid antibodies, thyroid function tests, anti-FcεRI, and anti-IgE antibodies.
- Treatments/prognosis
  - First attempt to identify and remove triggers.
  - Start with second-generation H1 antihistamine.
    - Can safely up-titrate dose to 4 times per day to control symptoms and flares for some agents.
  - If patient fails second-generation H1 antihistamine at 4 times per day, can add an H2 antagonist.
    - This step will not add much efficacy.
  - Omalizumab (anti-IgE monoclonal antibody) is FDA approved for chronic spontaneous urticaria (CSU). Dupilumab is also FDA approved to treat CSU.
    - If the patient has a history of asthma, an EpiPen should be prescribed as well when prescribing omalizumab.
  - Cyclosporine can be also used in severe, refractory cases of chronic urticaria.
- USMLE Board Review Pearls
  - Urticaria or "hives" is a very common symptom that can be seen as a symptom of another primary disease or process. On exams, watch out for the following: an allergic/anaphylactic reaction, a feature of a type I or

type III hypersensitivity reaction, side effect of sulfa drugs, and scombroid poisoning all causing hives.

- Look for pruritic, transient, edematous, pink/red papules, and plaques.
  - Due to release of histamine and prostaglandins from Mast cells and lesions last less than 24 hours.
- Episodes of chronic urticaria last longer than 6 weeks and is usually idiopathic.
- When a patient presents with acute urticaria, ask about new foods, medications, illnesses, and other environmental exposures (arthropod bite, heat, cold, vibration, sweat, water exposure).

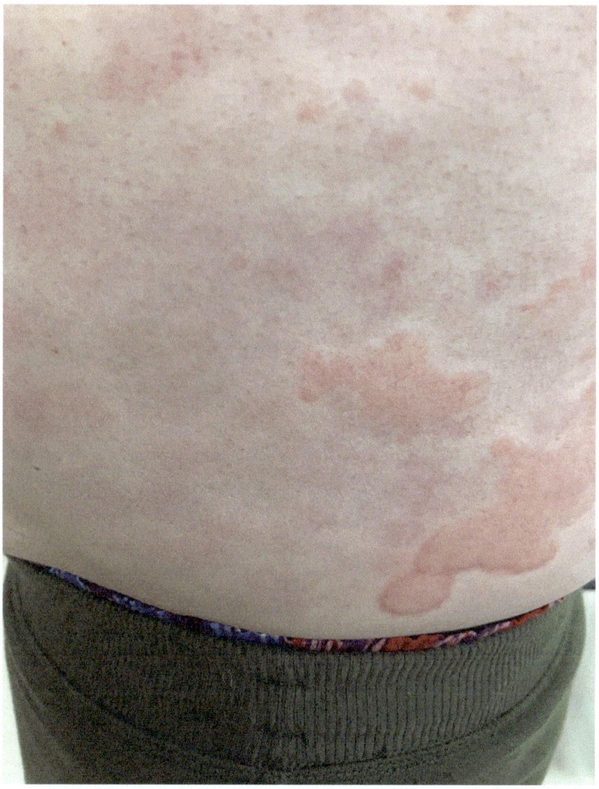

97. Urticarial vasculitis

- Morphology/clinical features
  - Same morphology as urticaria but lesions are fixed, last > 24 hours and burn/hurt rather than itch.

- Distribution
  - Favors the trunk and extremities.
- Etiology/pathogenesis
  - An idiopathic vasculitis driven by complement activation causing mast cell release of inflammatory mediators such as TNF that in turn increase the expression of ICAM on mast cells and E-selectin on endothelial cells.
- Internal sequelae/comorbidities
  - a/w autoimmune connective tissue diseases, **especially SLE** and Sjögren syndrome.
  - Musculoskeletal involvement is the most common extracutaneous manifestation of urticarial vasculitis.
- Laboratory testing
  - Histology will show a mild leukocytoclastic vasculitis.
  - Check ANA, ESR, C3, C4, C1q.
    - Patients with hypocomplementemia are much more likely to have systemic manifestations, such as GI, joint, or renal involvement!
- Treatments/prognosis
  - No randomized clinical trials have been performed to evaluate systemic therapy for this condition.
  - Start with oral corticosteroids but should not be used long term.
  - Can consider indomethacin, dapsone, colchicine, hydroxychloroquine, mycophenolate mofetil, rituximab, or anakinra.
  - Worse prognosis for the hypocomplementemic form.
  - Any clinician that sees urticaria with PIH should think of urticarial vasculitis.
- USMLE Board Review Pearls
  - Look for urticaria that does not resolve in 24 hours. The patient will complain of burning pain.
    - If you are unsure if the patient is describing urticaria or urticarial vasculitis, you can take a picture of a few lesions and have them return to clinic in 2–3 days to evaluate if the lesions have resolved.
  - The classic patient with this condition is a middle-aged woman with a history of SLE.
  - Schnitzler's syndrome = urticarial vasculitis, fevers, bone pain, arthralgia/arthritis, elevated ESR, and presence of IgM gammopathy.

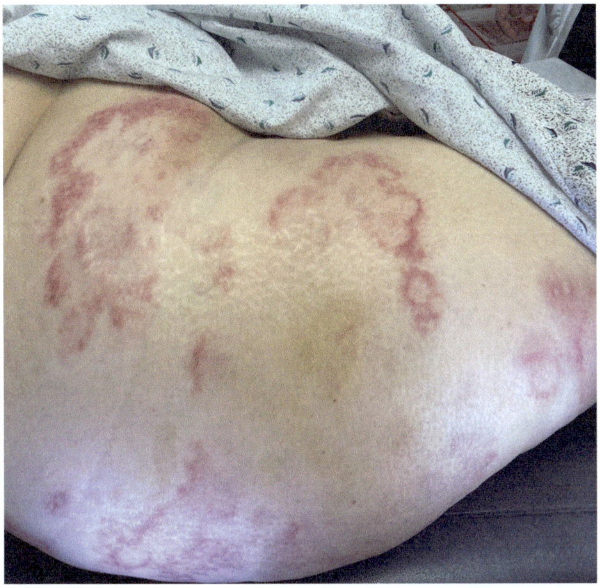

98. Varicella zoster

- Morphology/clinical features/distribution
  - Varicella—Cephalocaudal spread of characteristic lesions involving the head, trunk, and extremities described as vesicles on an erythematous base ("dew drops on rose petal") that become pustular, then crust over. Lesions are classically in different stages of development.
  - Herpes zoster—painful grouped vesicles on an erythematous base in a dermatomal pattern.
    - Vesicles will heal with a "scalloped border" or punched-out look.
    - Patients will usually complain of a painful or pruritic prodromal sensation before the characteristic eruption.
- Etiology/pathogenesis
  - The varicella zoster virus, also known as human herpesvirus 3 (HHV-3), causes varicella (chickenpox) and herpes zoster (shingles).
- Internal sequelae/comorbidities
  - In adults, varicella infection can cause severe pneumonia.
  - Varicella can cause serious neonatal and congenital infections.
  - Herpes zoster can lead to postherpetic neuralgia (chronic and debilitating pain).
  - Herpes zoster ophthalmicus can involve the eye leading to keratitis, uveitis, acute retinal necrosis, and visual loss.

    - Hutchinson's sign (involvement of the side and tip of nose): indicates disease of the external division of the V1 nasociliary branch.
        - Nasociliary nerve has three important divisions = infratrochlear (innervates nasal root, medial canthus) anterior ethmoidal (distal/ inferior half of central nose including dorsum, supratip, tip, and columella) and ciliary (corneal surface).
            - Thus, vesicles on the side or tip of the nose indicate involvement of the eye.
    - A patient with Hutchinson's sign needs evaluation by an ophthalmologist in addition to initiation of antiviral therapy.
        - If the patient does not have any ocular symptoms (redness, pain, change in vision, floaters), then they can be seen by outpatient ophthalmology as soon as possible.
        - If the patient is symptomatic, they need immediate evaluation in the Emergency Department by an ophthalmologist.
- Laboratory testing
    - PCR testing for VZV.
- Treatments/prognosis
    - Antiviral therapy with acyclovir, valacyclovir, or famciclovir.
        - A common treatment regimen for varicella and herpes zoster is valacyclovir 1 g TID for 7 days.
- USMLE Board Review Pearls
    - The varicella zoster virus (HHV-3) causes both varicella (chickenpox) and herpes zoster (shingles).
        - Shingles is a reactivation of the HHV-3 virus in a dermatomal distribution.
        - Disseminated shingles is possible in immunocompromised patients and is defined as >20 lesions outside of initial dermatome with or without visceral involvement.
    - Reye syndrome is a rare complication that may occur if a child takes aspirin to address the fever associated with varicella.
    - Varicella postexposure prophylaxis can be given for nonimmunized patients >12 months of age (immunoglobulin should be used for the immunocompromised, pregnant females and neonates and the vaccine for the immunocompetent).
    - Patients with varicella are infectious from 24 hours before eruption until lesions crust over.

- Human herpesvirus is an enveloped, double-stranded, linear virus.
- Know the eight types of HHV and the diseases that they cause.
    - HHV-1 = HSV-1
    - HHV-2 = HSV-2
    - HHV-3 = Varicella zoster virus
    - HHV-4 = Epstein–Barr virus
    - HHV-5 = cytomegalovirus (CMV)
    - HHV-6 / 7 = implicated in roseola, pityriasis rosea, and DRESS
    - HHV-8 = Kaposi sarcoma

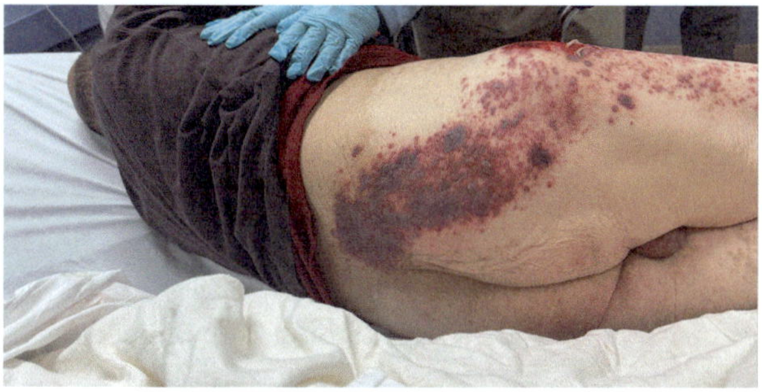

99. Verrucae (warts)

- Morphology/clinical features/distribution
    - Verruca vulgaris—classic description is a hyperkeratotic, papillomatous/warty ("cauliflower-like") papule with pinpoint black dots disrupting the normal dermatoglyphs (skin lines) on the fingers, dorsal hands, elbows, and knees but can be seen on the trunk and extremities.
    - Verruca plantaris/palmaris—thick, deep, broad, plaques with prominent black dots on palms and soles.
        - Myrmecial refers to the anthill appearance of some plantar warts.
    - Condyloma acuminatum ("genital wart")—genital/perianal skin.
        - Present as cauliflower-like skin-colored to brown papules.
    - Flat warts—dorsal hands, arms, and face in a linear array.
        - Present as skin-colored or pink to brown, relatively smooth surfaced, slightly elevated, flat-topped papules.
    - Warts can occur on mucosal skin.
        - Soft, pink/white, flat papules on mucosal skin.

- Etiology/pathogenesis
  - Human papillomavirus (HPV)
    - Verruca vulgaris/plantaris/palmaris = HPV 1, 2, 4.
    - Condyloma acuminata = HPV 6, 11, 16, 18.
    - Flat wart = HPV 3, 10.
- Internal sequelae/comorbidities
  - HPV infection may lead to cervical cancer.
  - Recurrent respiratory papillomatosis: papillomas of the airway due to HPV-6 and HPV-11.
    - Oral sex (genital-to-oral transmission) is increasingly being recognized as a possible risk factor.
- Laboratory testing
  - Can perform PCR for the presence of HPV.
- Treatments/prognosis
  - Shave excision, cryotherapy, imiquimod for condyloma acuminatum.
  - HPV vaccine for prevention (i.e., Gardasil or Cervarix).
- USMLE Board Review Pearls
  - High-risk HPV strains such as 16 and 18 can lead to SCC.
  - Warts are spread by direct contact.
  - Classic genital warts (condyloma acuminata) present as cauliflower-like skin-colored to brown papules on the genital or perianal skin and are caused by HPV 6 or 11.
    - **Must counsel all patients on the infectious nature of these warts and encourage barrier protection during intercourse and HPV vaccination. Females also need to be counseled on the risk of cervical cancer and follow-up with OBGYN for a pap smear.**
    - Genital warts can be treated by destructive measures (shave excision, cryosurgery) or with topical medications such as imiquimod.
      - Imiquimod works by binding toll-like receptor 7 (TLR-7), which leads to an increased immune response.
      - Side effects of this medication include itching and burning at site of application.

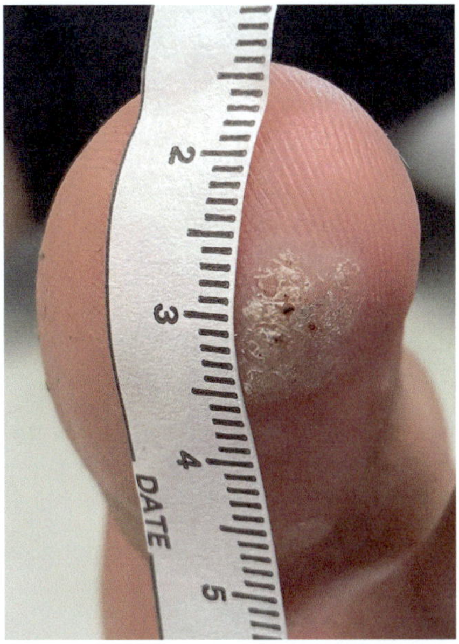

100. Vitiligo

- Morphology/clinical features
  - Depigmented, asymptomatic macules and patches.
- Distribution
  - Can occur anywhere but favors fingers, wrists, axillae, groin, genitals, and facial skin (around mouth/eyes).
- Etiology/pathogenesis
  - Genetic and nongenetic factors leading to autoimmune melanocyte destruction causing loss of pigment.
- Internal sequelae/comorbidities
  - a/w other autoimmune diseases.
    - Thyroid dysfunction is the most common association affecting up to 15% of patients.
- Laboratory testing
  - TSH
- Treatments/prognosis
  - Topical corticosteroids, topical calcineurin inhibitors, and phototherapy.

  - Topical ruxolitinib is the only FDA-approved therapy for re-pigmenting the skin.

- USMLE Board Review Pearls
  - Look for irregular patches and macules of complete depigmentation (stark white) on the hands and face. The patient will be asymptomatic.
  - Associated with other autoimmune conditions, especially thyroid disease.
    - If a patient does not have known thyroid disease, a thyroid function test should be ordered.
    - Type I DM is another common association.
  - Areas of depigmentation can be small (a few macules) to large patches and areas covering most of the body.
  - In lighter skin patients, the depigmentation may be more subtle.
    - A Wood's lamp may be used to help delineate the borders between depigmented and normal skin.
  - Mini-pulses of oral corticosteroids can be used for rapidly progressing disease.
  - Topical ruxolitinib, a JAK 1/2 inhibitor, is FDA approved for the treatment of vitiligo.
    - This is also FDA approved for atopic dermatitis.
  - Excimer laser (308nm) is another treatment option for vitiligo.

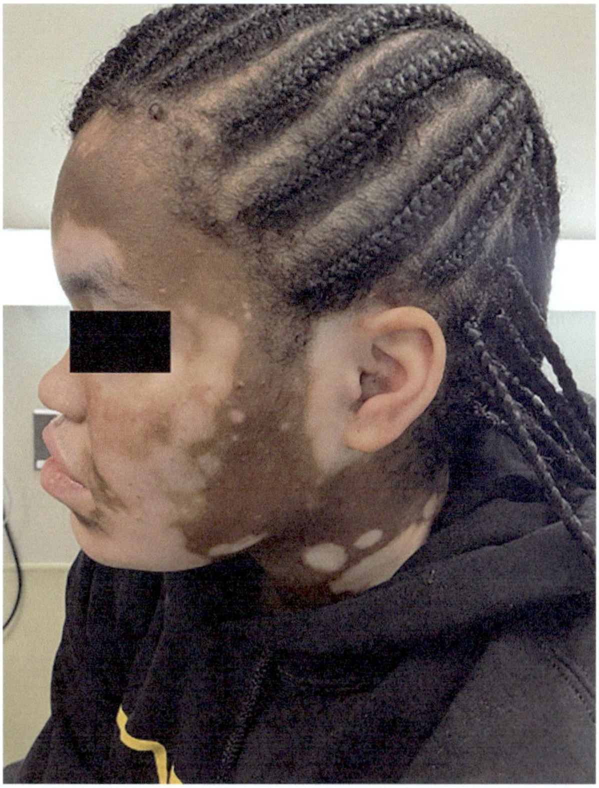

Chapter 4
Misnomers, Eponyms, and "Buzzwords/Phrases"

There are thousands of misnomers, eponyms, "buzzwords/phrases," confusing terms, sound-a-like terms, technical words, and alternative names for diagnoses in the field of dermatology. This section is by no means comprehensive or representative of all the examples above, but seeks to help the dermatology learner begin to comprehend and interpret the language of the field.

Misnomers

Misnomer	Explanation
Acanthosis nigricans	There is little to no acanthosis on histology
Adenoma sebeceum	These skin lesions, a/w tuberous sclerosis, are tiny angiofibromas and are not related to the sebaceous glands
Athlete's foot	Another term for tinea pedis. This condition commonly occurs in nonathletes
Axillary freckling	A sign a/w neurofibromatosis. By definition, freckles occur in sun-exposed areas and the axilla is non-sun exposed
Blue vitiligo	The color is actually a blue-gray, not strictly blue
Botryomycosis	This infection is due to *staph* bacteria and not fungal in nature despite having mycosis in the name
Bullous congenital ichthyosiform erythroderma (Bullous CIE)	This is not a true form of erythroderma
Buruli ulcer	This is an infection caused by mycobacteria, and there is no indication of an infectious nature in the name
Capillaritis	There is no clear evidence of vasculitis or inflammation of the capillaries on histology

(continued)

N. Brownstone, *The Ultimate Medical Student Guide to Dermatology*,
https://doi.org/10.1007/978-3-031-98765-6_4

Misnomer	Explanation
Chickenpox	This infection has nothing to do with chickens and cannot even cause infection in chickens
Cryotherapy	When this term is used for the treatment or destruction of skin lesions, it is a misnomer (the correct term is cryosurgery). Cryotherapy is the modulation of fat for cosmetic purposes or for the reduction of inflammation
Diffuse large B-cell lymphoma, leg type	A minority of cases present on skin outside of the leg
Digital myxoid cyst	Many of these cysts do not exhibit a lining histologically and therefore may be more appropriately termed pseudocysts
Dissecting cellulitis of scalp	The primary etiology of this condition is not infectious as the name "cellulitis" implies
Erythema toxicum neonatarum	This is a benign and transient neonatal rash, "toxicum" sounds dangerous and scary
Fibroepithelioma of Pinkus	While controversial, there is a general consensus that this skin lesion is actually a basal cell carcinoma and not a fibroepithelioma
Flat wart	These warts are slightly raised and are not completely flat
Granuloma faciale	There are no granulomas on histology
Granuloma fissuratum	Also known as acanthoma fissuratum, there are no granulomas on histology
Granuloma gluteale infantum	A form of diaper dermatitis. There are no granulomas on histology
Herpes gestationis	Another name for bullous pemphigoid of pregnancy; there is no association with herpes virus infection
Hot-comb alopecia	An older term for CCCA, while hot combs may contribute, recent research has moved away from this theory and hot combs certainly are not the only contributing factor
Impetigo herpetiformis	Another name for pustular psoriasis of pregnancy; there is no association with impetigo or herpes virus infection. This is a double misnomer!
Infantile myofibromatosis	This is a single lesion, and fibromatosis implies multiple lesions
Jock itch	Another term for tinea cruris. This condition commonly occurs in nonathletes
Kaposi sarcoma	Not a true sarcoma/malignancy in the traditional sense of the word
Keratosis follicularis	Another term for Darier disease; the keratotic papules are not necessarily follicular based
Liver spots	Liver spots are solar lentigines and have nothing to do with the liver or liver disease. They occur due to sun exposure
Lupus anticoagulant	These antibodies actually increase the risk of clotting
Lupus miliaris disseminatus faciei	This is a rosacea variant and has nothing to do with cutaneous lupus erythematosus
Lupus pernio	This is a variant of cutaneous sarcoidosis and has nothing to do with cutaneous lupus erythematosus
Lupus vulgaris	This is a form of cutaneous tuberculosis and has nothing to do with cutaneous lupus erythematosus

(continued)

Misnomer	Explanation
Lymphangiosarcoma	This is a type of angiosarcoma and is believed to arise from endothelial cells, not lymphatic cells
Malignant pustule	The term is used to describe a localized form of cutaneous anthrax and has nothing to do with cancer/malignancy
Microdermabrasion	This cosmetic treatment only impacts the epidermis and does not affect the dermis; a more correct term is "microepidermabrasion"
Molluscum fibrosum pendulum	Skin tag-like growths seen in tuberous sclerosis, Histopathologically, these lesions are characterized by epidermal papillomatosis with a central fibrovascular core and is not a form of molluscum contagiosum that is caused by a pox virus
Molluscum fibrosum gravidarum	This is a term used to describe skin tags that form in pregnancy and is not a form of molluscum contagiosum that is caused by a pox virus
Molluscoid pseudotumor	Growths that present as spongy outgrowths over sites of pressure, like elbows and knees in classical Ehlers–Danlos syndrome and is not a form of molluscum contagiosum that is caused by a pox virus
Mycosis fungoides	This is the most common form of cutaneous T-cell lymphoma and is not a fungal infection
Nevus depigmentosus	The skin lesion is hypopigmented, not depigmented
Nevus sebaceous	This is not a misnomer but is often incorrectly spelled as demonstrated here. The correct spelling is Nevus **Sebaceus**.
Nodulocystic acne	These acne lesions are not true cysts; they are dilated sebaceous glands
Palisaded encapsulated neuroma	This rare skin lesion that is neural in origin and does not appear palisaded or truly encapsulated on histology. A better term is the alternate name of solitary circumscribed neuroma
Papular urticaria	This is a term used to describe a bug bite, and it not a true form of urticaria
Pautrier's microabscess	This is a histological term used to describe a collection of lymphocytes; it is not infectious in nature and is not due to neutrophils as the name implies
Piezogenic papules	Piezogenic literally means pressure producing but these skin lesions are caused by pressure (i.e., piezogenic papules do not produce pressure)
Pretibial myxedema	While rare, pretibial myxedema can be seen outside of the pretibial area
Pubic lice	Pubic lice do not strictly affect the pubic area; it can also affect the eyebrows and eyelashes
Pyoderma gangrenosum	Pyoderma means "pus in the skin," and this is an immune-mediated skin disease that is not caused by an infection
Pyogenic granuloma	This single lesion is not due to an infection (despite pyogenic meaning "pus forming") and there are no granulomas on histology
Ringworm	This is another term for tinea corporis that is caused by a dermatophyte and not a worm

(continued)

Misnomer	Explanation
Rocky Mountain spotted fever	This infection is most commonly seen in the following states: North Carolina, Tennessee, Missouri, Arkansas, and Oklahoma and not in the Rocky Mountain States The Rocky Mountains are scattered across Arizona, Colorado, Idaho, Montana, Nevada, New Mexico, Utah, and Wyoming
Sebaceous cyst	Most nondermatologists will call any and all cysts (especially infundibular cysts) as sebaceous cysts. The only true sebaceous cyst is a steatocystoma
Seborrheic dermatitis	Seborrhea plays no part in the pathogenesis of the rash in most patients. A more correct term would be "dermatitis of the sebaceous areas"
Seborrheic keratosis	This common and benign skin lesion is actually derived from keratinocytes, not sebaceous glands
Senile purpura	While this condition impacts older patients, they are not all senile
Shagreen patch	This skin lesion is a plaque, not a patch (seen in tuberous sclerosis)
Sign of Leser-Trélat	This term originally described eruptive cherry angiomas but is now used to indicate eruptive seborrheic keratoses a/w internal malignancy
Tinea amiantacea	This is a term used to indicate very thick, white scales on the scalp. Psoriasis is the number 1 cause. It is not due to a dermatophyte. A more correct term is its alternate name, pityriasis amiantacea
Tinea cruris	"Cruris" is Latin for "of the leg" but tinea cruris is a term used to describe a dermatophyte infection of the groin
Tinea versicolor	This common and benign skin condition is caused by *Malassezia*, which is a type of yeast and not a dermatophyte as the name implies. A preferred name for this reason is its alternate name, pityriasis versicolor
Transient acantholytic dermatosis (Grover's disease)	In many cases, this condition is not transient at all and can persist
Trichomycosis axillaris	This skin infection, commonly seen on the axillary hair, is caused by bacteria and not a fungus as the name implies
Trichotillomania	This hair-pulling psychiatric disorder is not primarily a form of mania but classified as an obsessive-compulsive disorder in the DSM. A more correct term would be "trichotillooobsessivecompulsivedisorder"
Trumpeter's wart	This term describes a localized callus in trumpet players on the upper lip and is not due to HPV
Tumor of the follicular infundibulum	The name suggests this tumor originates from the follicular infundibulum, but histopathological studies indicate the cells show characteristics of the isthmus part of the hair follicle. By this definition, a seborrheic keratosis is a true "tumor of the follicular infundibulum." A more correct term for this tumor would be "tumor of isthmic cell differentiation"
Urticaria pigmentosa	This is a form of mastocytosis and not urticaria
Weathering nodules	Double misnomer! These are papules, not nodules, and "weathering" refers to the process of deterioration of rocks, soil, minerals through contact with water, atmospheric gases, sunlight, and biological organisms. A more correct name would be "sun exposure papules"

Eponyms

Eponym	Meaning
Acrodermatitis Continua of Hallopeau	A subtype of psoriasis characterized by pustules and bony destruction of the distal phalanges
Angel Kiss	Nevus simplex
Arnold's nerve	The auricular branch of the Vagus nerve
Asboe-Hansen sign	A blister that extends into nearby unblistered skin when pressure is applied to the top of the blister. Seen in TEN
Athlete's foot	Tinea pedis
Atrophoderma of Pasini and Pierini	Subtype of morphea
Auspitz sign	Small bleeding pinpoint areas when the skin scales of psoriasis are scraped away
Baker's itch	Caused by grain mite (*Acarus siro*)
Barnett's sign	Visible and palpable tight band over platysma in the hyperextended neck a/w scleroderma
Barraquer–Simons syndrome	Acquired partial Lipodystrophy
Bart syndrome	A type of epidermolysis bullosa a/w localized absence of skin often on the limbs
Beau's lines	Transverse depressions in the nail plate that are commonly caused by a stressful event
Bednar tumor	A pigmented DFSP
Berardinelli–Seip syndrome	Congenital generalized Lipodystrophy
Berliner sign	Eyelid edema in children, which can make their eyes appear heavy, droopy, or sleepy that is seen in roseola
Bier spots	Angiospastic macules due to localized vasoconstriction
Biett's sign/scale	Refers to the peripheral scaling around the papules and plaques seen in the eruption of secondary syphilis
Bloch–Sulzberger disease	Incontinentia pigmenti
Bohn nodules	Milia on the alveolar ridge of a newborn
Bolognia sign	Melanocytic nevi with eccentric foci of hyperpigmentation
Bourneville–Pringle disease	Tuberous sclerosis
Bowen's disease	Also known as squamous cell carcinoma in situ
Bruch's membrane	A thin, five-layered membrane in the eye that separates the retina from the choroid. Relevant to dermatologists because patients with pseudoxanthoma elasticum can get calcification of this membrane leading to vision loss
Casal's necklace	An exam finding in pellagra characterized by well-demarcated hyperpigmentation around the neck
Chiclero's ulcer	Cutaneous leishmaniasis located on the ear
Christ–Siemens–Touraine syndrome	Hypohidrotic ectodermal dysplasia

(continued)

Eponym	Meaning
Clark nevus	Dysplastic or atypical nevus
Clouston disease	Hidrotic ectodermal dysplasia
Crow's sign	Characteristic of neurofibromatosis type 1, appears as freckling in the armpits or groin
Cullen's sign	Superficial edema and bruising in the subcutaneous fatty tissue around the umbilicus a/w acute pancreatitis
Cupid's bow	Double curve of the human upper lip which resembles the bow of Cupid, the Roman God of love
Cushing syndrome	Hypercortisolism leading to numerous skin and systemic signs and symptoms
Darier disease	Also known as keratosis follicularis
Darier's sign	Rubbing a lesion of mastocytoma causes urtication, flare, swelling and sometimes blister formation due to release of histamine
Darwin's tubercle	Congenital ear condition that often presents as a thickening on the helix at the junction of the upper and middle thirds
Degos acanthoma	Clear/pale cell acanthoma
Degos disease	Malignant atrophic papulosis, also referred to as Köhlmeier–Degos disease
Dennie–Morgan lines	Small creases or folds that appear under the lower eyelid a/w atopic diathesis
Doucas and Kapetanakis	Describes the eczematid-like eruption of pigmented purpuric dermatosis
Dowling-Meara	Epidermolysis bullosa simplex—generalized severe
du Bois sign	Characterizes the condition of a shortened fifth finger as a symptom of congenital syphilis or Down syndrome
Duhring disease	Dermatitis herpetiformis
Duncan's dirty dermatosis	Terra firma-forme dermatosis also known as retention hyperkeratosis
Epstein pearls	Milia on the hard palate of newborns
Erb's point	Describes the point on the posterior border of the SCM muscle, approximately 2–3 cm above the clavicle, overlying the transverse process of the sixth cervical vertebra, where the four superficial branches of the cervical plexus—the greater auricular, lesser occipital, transverse cervical, and supraclavicular nerves—emerge from behind the muscle
Favre–Racouchot syndrome	Multiple open comedones on sun-damaged skin
Finkelstein disease	Acute hemorrhagic edema of infancy
Fitzpatrick skin type	A classification system that estimates how skin reacts to ultraviolet (UV) light, named after American dermatologist Thomas Fitzpatrick, MD, PhD. This is sometimes used incorrectly to describe a patient's skin tone
Fong disease	Nail-patella syndrome
Forchheimer's spots	A type of enathem seen as tiny red spots on the soft palate seen in Rubella
Fordyce spots	Ectopic sebaceous glands on the lips/oral mucosa
Fox–Fordyce disease	Apocrine miliaria
Frank's sign	Diagonal crease in the earlobe that runs from the tragus to the rear edge of the auricle at a 45° angle a/w cardiovascular disease

(continued)

Eponym	Meaning
Frey's syndrome	Auriculotemporal syndrome characterized by hyperhidrosis and localized flushing with salivation, aka "gustatory sweating"
Friar tuck sign	A pattern of hair loss seen in trichotillomania
Goltz syndrome	Focal dermal hypoplasia
Gorlin syndrome	Basal cell nevus syndrome
Gottron's papules	Small, flat, red, or purple papules that appear on the knuckles of the fingers, elbows, or knees seen in patients with dermatomyositis
Gougerot–Carteaud syndrome	Confluent and reticulated papillomatosis (CARP)
Grey Turner's sign	A rare sign that indicates internal bleeding in the abdomen and is characterized by bruising or discoloration on the flanks or lower back
Grocer's itch	Caused by Cheese mite (*Glyciphagus*)
Grover's disease	Transient acantholytic dermatosis
Gougerot and Blum	Describes the lichenoid variant of pigmented purpuric dermatosis
Hailey–Hailey disease	Benign familial pemphigus
Hamilton–Norwood scale	Used to classify the stages of male androgenetic alopecia
Hansen's disease	Leprosy
Hashimoto–Pritzker disease	Congenital self-healing reticulohistiocytosis
Heck's disease	Focal epithelial hyperplasia caused by HPV 13 and 32
Henderson–Patterson bodies	Characteristic intracytoplasmic inclusion bodies seen histologically in molluscum contagiosum
Higoumenakis' sign	Enlargement of the sternal end of the clavicle, frequently observed in patients with late congenital syphilis
Hinderers' lines	Indicates the appropriate target for cheek filler injections
Hoagland sign	Early and transient bilateral upper lid edema occurring in patients with mononucleosis
Hutchinson's sign (nail)	Pigmentation on the proximal nail fold that can be a/w nail melanoma
Hutchinson's sign (nose)	Vesicles on the tip of the nose in herpes zoster that usually indicate ocular involvement (herpes zoster ophthalmicus)
Hutchinson's teeth	Smaller, wider-spaced teeth with notching seen in congenital syphilis
Hutchinson's triad	Triad in late congenital syphilis consisting of notched incisors, interstitial keratitis, and eighth cranial nerve deafness
Jackson–Lawler syndrome	Pachyonychia congenita type II
Kawasaki disease	Mucocutaneous lymph node syndrome characterized by fever, vasculitis, red eyes, lymphadenopathy, rash, and cardiac complications
Klein solution	A type of tumescent solution consisting of lidocaine, epinephrine, saline, and sodium bicarbonate that is used in liposuction and other procedures
Kligman's formula	A triple combination topical consisting of hydroquinone, tretinoin, and topical corticosteroid. Named after American dermatologist Alfred Kligman, MD, PhD

(continued)

Eponym	Meaning
Köbberling–Dunnigan syndrome	Familial partial lipodystrophy
Koebner phenomenon	Describes the appearance of new skin lesions of a preexisting dermatosis on areas of cutaneous injury in otherwise healthy skin
Koenen tumor	Periungual or subungual fibroma seen in tuberous sclerosis
Koo–Brownstone staging system	The first and only staging system developed to stage/manage patients who present with dermatological delusions. Created by and named after American dermatologists John Koo, MD and Nicholas Brownstone, MD (who is also the author of this book!)
Koplik spots	Small, white, or bluish-white spots that appear on the inside of the cheeks seen in measles
Kunze–Riehm syndrome	Michelin tire baby syndrome
Kyrle disease	Acquired perforating dermatosis
Lawrence syndrome	Acquired generalized Lipodystrophy
Lederhosen disease	Plantar fibromatosis
Lindsay's nails	Half and half nails a/w renal disease (half of the nail is white and half is reddish/brown)
Lipschitz ulcer	A rare, idiopathic, nonsexually transmitted type of genital ulcer that usually affects young women and adolescents (viral infections such as EBV may play a role)
Lisch nodules	Iris hamartomas seen in neurofibromatosis type 1
Louis–Bar syndrome	Ataxia telangiectasia
Lucio phenomenon	A rare reactional state seen in cases of diffuse lepromatous leprosy primarily seen in Mexico and Central America
Ludwig scale	Used to classify the stages of female androgenetic alopecia
Majocchi's granuloma	Deep and persistent suppurative and granulomatous folliculitis (hair follicle infection) caused by fungal infection
Martoll ulcer	A leg ulcer a/w hypertension
Melkerson–Rosenthal syndrome	Cheilitis granulomatosa characterized by recurrent or persistent orofacial edema (facial and lip edema), fissured tongue, and relapsing, unilateral or bilateral peripheral facial nerve paralysis
Mikulicz's disease	A condition involving the enlargement of the lacrimal and salivary glands seen in Sjögren's syndrome
Mohs surgery	A specialized type of skin cancer surgery named after American Surgeon Frederic E. Mohs, MD
Monsel's solution	Ferric subsulfate, a topical hemostatic agent
Montgomery tubercles	Ectopic sebaceous glands on the areola or nipple
Morbihan's disease	Solid facial edema (variant of rosacea)
Morgellons disease	An unofficial term for Delusions of Parasitosis
Mucha–Habermann disease	Another name for pityriasis lichenoides et varioliformis acuta (PLEVA)
Muehrcke's nails	Multiple transverse whitish bands, parallel to the lunula seen in hypoalbuminemia and chemotherapy

(continued)

Eponym	Meaning
Myerson nevus	A melanocytic nevus surrounded by eczema
Nagashima disease	Prurigo pigmentosa
Nagayama spots	A characteristic feature of roseola characterized by red spots on the soft palate and uvula
Nikolsky sign	A dermatological sign that occurs when the top layer of skin separates from the lower layers when the skin is rubbed or sheared that is seen in pemphigus vulgaris, TEN, SSSS
Nonne–Milroy syndrome	Hereditary congenital lymphedema
Osler node	Painful, red, raised lesions found on the hands and feet a/w a number of conditions, including infective endocarditis
Pastia lines	Pink or red lines formed from confluent petechiae in skin creases seen in scarlet fever
Pinkus tumor	A type of basal cell carcinoma (although the malignant nature of this lesion is controversial)
Pitanguy's line	Pitanguy's line is the classic reference line for the general path of the frontal branch of the facial nerve within the temporal regions. This landmark is an imaginary line drawn from the base of the tragus to 1.5 cm above the ipsilateral eyebrow
Queen Anne's sign/ sign of Hertoghe	Thinning or loss of the outer third of the eyebrows a/w hypothyroidism or atopic dermatitis
Quelprud's nodule	A small, prominent cartilaginous bump on the back of the ear. Named after Thordar Quelprud, a Norwegian geneticist
Rieger flap	Dorsal nasal flap used to repair Mohs defects around the nose and eye
Riehl melanosis	A type of hyperpigmented contact dermatitis
Romaña's sign	A symptom of acute Chagas disease which causes swelling of the eyelid
Rosai–Dorfman disease	Sinus histiocytosis with massive lymphadenopathy
Rowell syndrome	An erythema multiforme-like presentation of SCLE
Rumpel–Leede sign	Ecchymoses and petechiae that appear after pressure is released from a tourniquet or BP cuff due to broken capillaries
Russell's sign	Defined as calluses on the knuckles or back of the hand due to repeated self-induced vomiting over long periods of time, secondary to eating disorders such as Bulimia
Samitz's sign	Nail-fold telangiectasias and ragged cuticles seen in Dermatomyositis
Schaumann body	Rounded laminated basophilic inclusions seen in diseases such as sarcoidosis that represents degenerating lysosomes
Seabather's eruption	Eruption under covered areas after swimming in salt water due to *Edwardsiella lineata* (sea anemone) and *Linuche unguiculata* (thimble jellyfish)
Senear–Usher syndrome	Pemphigus erythematosus
Shulman syndrome	Eosinophilic fasciitis
Shuster sign	Scarring of the concha secondary to discoid lupus erythematosus
Sign of Leser-Trélat	Sudden appearance of a large number of seborrheic keratoses a/w malignancy
Sipple syndrome	Multiple endocrine neoplasia type 2A

(continued)

Eponym	Meaning
Sister Mary Joesph nodule	A palpable nodule found in the umbilicus that indicates metastasis from a GI malignancy
Sneddon–Wilkinson disease	Subcorneal pustular dermatosis
Spider nevus	Nevus araneus
St. Anthony's fire	Refers to either erysipelas or ergotism
Stensen's duct	Parotid duct
Stewart–Treves syndrome	Angiosarcoma arising in chronic lymphedema
Stork bite	Nevus simplex on the posterior neck
Sutton nevus	Halo nevus
Swimmer's itch	Cercarial dermatitis characterized by eruption on uncovered skin after swimming in fresh water
Terry's nails	Leukonychia of the entire nail (sparing distal 1-2 mm) a/w liver cirrhosis
Tokelau	Tinea imbricata
Triton tumor	Rare, aggressive subtype of a malignant peripheral nerve sheath tumor
Tyndall effect	A phenomenon that occurs when visible light passes through a medium with irregularities, causing short-wavelength light to scatter and reflect back to the observer
Tyson glands	Ectopic sebaceous glands on the male genitalia
Urbach–Weithe disease	Lipoid proteinosis
Vampire disease	Refers to porphyrias; Dracula was thought to suffer from a porphyria
Von Recklinghausen disease	Neurofibromatosis type 1 (NF1)
Von Zumbusch psoriasis	Generalized pustular psoriasis
Walzel sign	A type of livedo reticularis associated with acute or chronic pancreatitis
Weber–Cockayne syndrome	Epidermolysis bullosa simplex—localized
Wermer syndrome	Multiple endocrine neoplasia type I
Whitfield's ointment	An acidic ointment used for the topical treatment of dermatophytosis, original ointment contained 3% salicylic acid and 6% benzoic acid in a vehicle, such as lanolin or petrolatum. Named after Arthur Whitfield, MD, a British dermatologist
Wickham's striae	Fine white or gray lines/dots that appear on the top of papules/plaques and oral mucosal lesions of lichen planus
Winterbottom sign	Posterior triangle cervical lymphadenopathy seen in trypanosomiasis
Wood's lamp	Named after physicist Robert Williams Wood, this is a type of ultraviolet light source used to detect fluorescence in various material (peak wavelength around 365 nm)
Woronoff ring	White, ring-shaped area of hypopigmentation that can appear around regressing psoriasis papules/plaques
Zinsser–Engman–Cole syndrome	Dyskeratosis congenita
Zitelli flap	A modification of the bilobed flap used to reconstruct nasal defects after Mohs surgery, named after American dermatologist/Mohs surgeon John Zitelli, MD
Zoon's balanitis	A chronic inflammatory skin condition that affects the genital mucosa

"Buzzwords"/"Buzz Phrases"

Buzzword/phrase	Meaning
Allergic salute	The act of rubbing or wiping the nose upwards with the fingers, palm, or back of the hand, resulting in a hyperpigmented horizontal line or crease across the lower part of the nose bridge seen in patients with allergies
Allergic shiner	Dark circles that appear under the eyes a/w sinus congestion and allergies
Arborizing vessels	Vessel pattern seen on dermoscopy characteristic of basal cell carcinoma
Ash leaf macule	Ash leaf-shaped white macules seen in tuberous sclerosis
Ashy dermatosis	Erythema dyschromicum perstans
Asteroid body	Microscopic, star-shaped structures that can be found in the cytoplasm of giant cells in a variety of diseases such as sarcoidosis, represents degenerated collagen
Baby doll hairs	Polytrichia, in which multiple hairs emerge from a single follicular opening that leads to tufting, seen in CCCA
Bag of worms	Description of a plexiform neurofibroma (in my opinion after palpating a few of these lesions, I would recommend changing the buzzword to "water-ballon" as it feels more like this to me than a bag of worms)
Bathing suit distribution	Lesions or rash involving the area of the skin covered by the bathing suit bottoms which can be seen with mycosis fungodies, Seabather's eruption, and Fabry's disease
Bilateral lower extremity cellulitis	This is usually never due to frank cellulitis but is usually a description of lipodermatosclerosis
Black fever	Visceral leishmaniasis
Blue gray veil	Dermatoscopic finding in melanoma
Blueberry muffin baby	This term was originally used to describe the skin manifestations of congenital rubella
Breakfast, lunch, and dinner sign	Bite marks clustered in small groups, spaced just a few centimeters apart characteristic of an arthropod assault. Arthropods usually bite a few times in a row (can also be referred to as breakfast, lunch, snack and dinner sign if there are 4 arthropod bites in a row or group)
Buffalo hump	Also known as a dorsocervical fat pad, a buildup of fat in the back of the neck that can cause the shoulders to appear humped, seen in Cushing syndrome
Bullseye rash	Erythema migrans
Bunny lines	Wrinkles that appear on the nose during certain facial expressions
Butterfly rash	Eruption of ACLE on the face sparing the nasolabial folds
Butterfly sign	Excoriations and prurigo nodules sparing the area of the back where a patient cannot reach
Buttonhole sign	Ability to press a soft skin lesion, like a neurofibroma, into the underlying tissue, creating a depression that resembles pushing a finger through a buttonhole. The lesion can be pushed into the skin and then pops back out when pressure is released. Also appreciated in anetoderma
Café-au-lait macules	Flat, pigmented macules/patches on the skin that are usually light to dark brown in color a/w neurofibromatosis type 1 (NF1)

(continued)

Buzzword/phrase	Meaning
Café noir spots	Larger and darkly pigmented patches/macules that are frequently observed in patients who have Noonan syndrome with multiple lentigines (previously referred to as LEOPARD syndrome)
Candy cane nails	Alternating red/white nail streaks seen in Darier disease
Carnauba wax	Describes the PPK seen in PRP
Carpet tack spines	In DLE, characteristic lesions are well-defined erythematous plaques with partially adherent scales entering a patulous follicle. When the scale is removed, its undersurface shows keratotic plugs that had occupied follicles
Cathectic dwarfism	Cockayne syndrome
Cauliflower lesion	Describes the morphology of a condyloma acuminatum
Cayenne pepper spots	Describes the pinpoint petechiae seen in Schamberg disease or any other PPD
Chicken skin	Keratosis pilaris
Chocolate Chip Cookie lesion	Nevus spilus
Christmas tree rash	Describes the morphology of pityriasis rosea following skin lines on the back
Cliff drop sign	Describes the subtle depression seen in lesions of Atrophoderma of Pasini and Pierini
Coast of Maine macule	Café au lait lesions with rough, jagged borders that are seen in McCune–Albright syndrome
Cobblestone mucosa	Characteristic feature of Darier disease, Crohn's disease, and Cowden syndrome
Confetti macules	Hypomelanotic macules seen in tuberous sclerosis
Copper-colored acral lesions/Nickel and dime lesions	Describes the morphology of secondary syphilis
Coral beads	Papules seen around the nail fold in multicentric reticulohistiocytosis
Coral red glow	Fluorescent pattern/color seen in erythrasma due to coproporphyrin III under a Wood's lamp
Corkscrew hairs	A characteristic change in hairs that is seen in scurvy
Cornflake scale	Describes the loose scale seen in pemphigus foliaceus
Cracks in the porcelain	Describes the dry, cracked look of asteatotic eczema
Crateriform lesion	Describes the morphology of a keratoacanthoma
Crow's feet	Periocular wrinkles
Crowe's sign	Presence of axillary freckling in patients with neurofibromatosis type I
Crown of jewel blisters	Groups of small blisters in an annular configuration seen in linear IgA bullous disease
Crown vessels	Dermoscopic pattern seen in sebaceous gland hyperplasia
Deck chair sign	A clinical pattern where skin folds are selectively spared during an erythematous eruption, seen in papuloerythroderma of Ofuji
Dermatomal rash/ eruption	Herpes zoster
Dewdrops on a rose petal	Describes the morphology of herpesvirus infection, seen in chickenpox

(continued)

Buzzword/phrase	Meaning
Dimple sign	Dermatological sign that appears when the skin around a dermatofibroma is squeezed, causing a central depression
Dolly Parton sign	"Too many lymphocytes for too little spongiosis." Describes the histological pattern seen in the epidermis of mycosis fungoides
Double-covered area	Erythematous scaly plaques involving the buttocks that are covered by both the underwear and pants, characteristic of mycosis fungoides
Double edge scale	In the context of Netherton syndrome refers to the characteristic appearance of ichthyosis linearis circumflexa
Doughnut pustule	Describes the morphology of the lesions seen in Mpox (preferred term for Monkeypox according the World Health Organization)
Dry River Bed	Linear grooving or depressions (due to underlying veins) seen in eosinophilic fasciitis
Dufourmentel flap	A modification of the rhomboid flap named after French plastic surgeon, Claude Dufourmentel
Exclamation point hairs	Describes the morphology of the hairs seen in alopecia areata, hairs are narrower at the base versus the distal tip
Football-shaped vesicles	Describes the classic appearance of the vesicles seen in hand, foot, and mouth disease
Frog spawn lesions	Lymphangioma circumscriptum
Geographic tongue	Benign migratory glossitis
Geometric ulcers/ geometric burns	Indicates either dermatitis artefacta or abuse of the skin
Golden/rust-colored patch	Lichen aureus
Gorlin's sign	The ability of patients with Ehlers–Danlos syndrome to touch the tip of the nose with the tip of their tongue. 10% of the normal population and 50% of patients with Ehlers–Danlos can achieve this
Hair collar sign	A marker of cranial dysraphism, including encephalocele, meningocele, and heterotopic brain tissue
Hairy palm sign	It is a characteristic histopathological finding seen in prurigo nodularis/ LSC, where there is a presence of thick compact orthohyperkeratosis with folliculosebaceous units
Herald patch	Describes the initial larger plaque seen in the eruption of pityriasis rosea
Herringbone pattern	Describes the histology of a DFSP
Hoarse cry	Seen in infants with lipoid proteinosis or epidermolysis bullosa
Holster sign rash	Erythema of the lateral hips seen in dermatomyositis
Honey-colored crusts	Scaling/crusting seen in impetigo (note that contact dermatitis can also have this feature but this is due to exuberant spongiosis and not an infection)
Honeycomb PPK	Describes the appearance of the PPK seen in Vohwinkel syndrome
Hound dog facies	Describes the facial features seen in Cutis laxa
Inverted fir tree pattern	Pattern seen in median canaliform nail dystrophy
Inverted wine bottle appearance	Describes the findings seen in lipodermatosclerosis (if you are feeling particularly fancy, you can use the term "inverted champagne bottle")
Islands of sparing	Areas of normal skin that appear within the scaly plaques of pityriasis rubra pilaris

(continued)

Buzzword/phrase	Meaning
Keto diet rash	Prurigo pigmentosa
Kissing lesions	Describes rash involving adjacent/touching areas that is seen in Zoon balanitis
Knife-like ulcers	A cutaneous manifestation of Crohn's disease characterized by sharp, linear ulcerations in the groin/genital region
Knuckle pads	A localized form of fibromatosis on the dorsal hands
Leaves of three, let it be	A rhyme that helps to identify Poison Ivy
Lesions in different stages	Chickenpox
Lesions in the same stage	Smallpox
Limberg flap	Another term for a rhomboid flap
Mask of pregnancy	Melasma
Matchbox sign	Describes a behavior seen in patients with delusions of parasitosis who bring in Ziploc bags with hair, dirt, dust, and skin cells to prove they have a parasitic infection
Mechanics hands	Describes the roughed, hyperkeratotic, and scaly hands seen in antisynthetase syndrome
Mexican beer drinker dermatitis	A generalized form of phytophotodermatitis
Micaceous scale	Describes the thick, white scale of psoriasis
Moccasin distribution	Describes the distribution of tinea pedis on the bottom and sides of the foot
Moon facies	An increase in the adipose tissue of the face, seen in Cushing syndrome
Moth eaten alopecia	A type of hair loss that appears as multiple small, irregularly shaped patches on the scalp that is a/w syphilis
Mousy order	Odor in the breath, skin, urine, or ear wax a/w phenylketonuria
Necklace of Venus	White spots on the side of the neck a/w syphilis
Nodules in a plaque	Describes the palpation of a DFSP
Oil drop spots	Nail discoloration seen in psoriasis
Pain out of proportion to exam	A key clinical finding that strongly suggests the presence of necrotizing fasciitis
Painful chancre	Chancroid
Painless chancre	Syphilis
Pearly lesion	Basal cell carcinoma
Pearly penile papules	Angiofibromas usually seen on the penile corona
Peau d'orange	A term used to describe a symptom in which the skin becomes thick and pitted, with a texture and appearance similar to that of an orange peel. Can be seen in various conditions such as carcinoma en cuirasse, nephrogenic systemic fibrosis, eosinophilic fasciitis, scleredema, pretibial myxedema, and granuloma faciale
Pencil-in-cup deformity	Bone destruction pattern of the fingers seen on X-rays that is most commonly associated with severe psoriatic arthritis
Pinch purpura	Purpuric macules and ecchymoses, especially in the periorbital area, develop with minor trauma because of fragility from amyloid deposition seen in systemic amyloidosis

(continued)

Buzzword/phrase	Meaning
Plucked chicken skin	Wrinkled skin seen in pseudoxanthoma elasticum
Popsicle rash	A form of cold panniculitis seen on the cheek of a child
Punched out lesions	Ulcerations seen in eczema herpeticum
Purple, planar, polygonal, pruritic papules	Describes lichen planus
Question mark repair	Describes the appearance of the final suture line after performing a rhomboid flap
Racoon eyes	Periorbital erythema and edema seen in neonatal lupus
Ram horn nail	Onychogryphosis
Raspberry papillomas	Lesions seen around the mouth in patients with focal dermal hypoplasia
Red hourglass	Pattern seen on the abdomen (ventral surface) of a black widow spider
Red man syndrome	An infusion-related reaction caused by vancomycin
Red touches yellow kills a fellow	A rhyme to help remember the colors of the venomous coral snake. Coral snakes possess one of the most potent venoms of any North American snake
Ringworm	Tinea corporis
Rippled potato chip	Describes the appearance of macular amyloidosis
Rippled seafloor appearance	Describes the appearance of lichen amyloidosis
Rock hard lesion	Describes the palpation of a cutaneous granular cell tumor
Rodent ulcer	An ulceration caused by basal cell carcinoma
Rope sign	Thick indurated inflammatory cord-like structure that extends from the lateral trunk to the axillae, said to be a classic finding of interstitial granulomatous dermatitis
Rose spots	A rash that appears on the trunk in patients with typhoid fever
Salt and pepper dyspigmentation	Vitiligo-like depigmentation with retained pigment around hair follicles seen characteristically in scleroderma
Sandal-like PPK	PPK characteristic of PR
Satellite pustules	Small, itchy, blister-like lesions that appear near a larger, primary lesion, usually in skin folds seen in *Candida* infections
Saxophone penis	A term used to describe a condition where the penis twists along its long axis, causing it to resemble a saxophone a/w hidradenitis suppurativa or inflammatory bowel disease
Scalloped ulcer/border	An irregular, wavy edge of an ulcer, resembling the scalloped pattern of a seashell, often seen in conditions like herpesvirus infections
Serpiginous border	Describes the wavy and uneven border of tinea corporis
Shawl sign rash	A flat, reddened area that appears on the upper back, shoulders, and posterior neck seen in dermatomyositis
Simian crease	Also known as a single palmar crease or transverse palmar crease, seen in Down syndrome
Slapped cheeks	Bilateral erythema of the cheeks seen in Parvovirus B19 infection
Splash of paint lesion	Describes the morphology of a nevus depigmentosus
Starburst pattern	Describes the pattern of Reed nevus on dermoscopy
Starfish-shaped keratoses	Papules seen in patients with Vohwinkel syndrome

(continued)

Buzzword/phrase	Meaning
Strawberries and cream	Describes the appearance of extramammary Paget disease due to scattered areas of white scale and erosions on a deep red plaque
Strawberry gums	Describes the gingival hemorrhage with a friable micropapillary surface seen in granulomatosis with polyangiitis (old term is Wegener granulomatosis)
Strawberry tongue	A tongue that's red with large bumps that look like the skin of a strawberry that can be seen in scarlet fever, toxic shock syndrome, or Kawasaki disease
Stuck on papule	Describes the appearance of a seborrheic keratosis
Swarm of bees	Describes the lymphocytic infiltrate seen in alopecia areata on histology
Tapioca vesicles	Describes the appearance of the vesicles seen in dyshidrotic eczema
Target lesions	Classically describes the morphology of erythema multiforme
Teeter totter sign	A dermatological sign that indicates a pilomatrixoma, when pressure is applied to one end of the lesion, the other end elevates
The itch that rashes	Describes the severe pruritus that is a/w atopic dermatitis
Thinker's lines	Wrinkles in the glabella, also known as "eleven lines"
Thread like peripheral scale	Describes the peripheral, thin scale of a porokeratosis
Thumbprint purpura	Seen around the umbilicus in a Strongyloidiasis infection
Toad skin	Describes the skin change that is seen in phrynoderma
Tobacco patch sign	A localized area of skin discoloration or irritation, usually appearing as a red, irritated patch, where a nicotine patch has been applied
Trailing scale	Characteristic scale of erythema annulare centrifugum, can be seen in many other conditions as well
Triangular lunula	A pathognomonic finding in nail-patella syndrome is the presence of triangular-shaped lunula
Two feet-one hand rash	Dermatophyte infection of both feet and one hand
Ugly duckling lesion	A nevus that does not resemble other nevi is more likely to be suspicious of melanoma
Undermined, violaceous border	Describes the border of an ulcer due to pyoderma gangrenosum
Unhappy clown	Describes the facial appearance of a child with staph scaled skin syndrome (SSSS)
V-sign	Confluent V-shaped macular violaceous erythema on the anterior neck and chest in patients with dermatomyositis
Violin-shaped marking	Pattern on the cephalothorax of a brown recluse spider
Waxy papules	Describes the lesions seen in scleromyxedema
Webster flap	A modification of the rhomboid flap which uses a more acute angle
White islands in a sea of red	Dengue infection can cause a confluent, non-blanching erythematous rash with macules and patches of normal skin within the erythema
Woodgrain rash	Describes the characteristic appearance of erythema gyratum repens
Wrinkled cigarette paper	Describes the appearance of lichen sclerosus
Ziti and meatballs	Describes the KOH prep findings in tinea versicolor (represents hyphae and spores)

Chapter 5
The Ultimate Skin Care Secret

As a physician, and especially as a dermatologist, you are going to be bombarded with hundreds of skincare products claiming to slow or reverse skin aging.

You will see these products in the pharmacy, in the grocery store, in magazines, on billboards, in movies, on the Internet, on social media, on TV, and promoted by celebrities who we all idolize.

Your patients will ask about these products and will want to know … does it really work? Despite all of these products out there, below you find the two most important skin care secrets that will lead to healthier and better-looking skin throughout a lifetime. They are

1. Don't smoke
2. Wear sunscreen

If practiced throughout a lifetime, these two skin care principles will be more effective than any product currently on the market aimed at treating the sequelae of skin aging.

I hope you have enjoyed this book and hope that what you have learned here will both motivate you to explore dermatology further and improve patient care in your career. Good luck!

N. Brownstone, *The Ultimate Medical Student Guide to Dermatology*,
https://doi.org/10.1007/978-3-031-98765-6_5

Suggested Reading

1. https://evolve.elsevier.com/cs/product/9780702082252?role=student
2. https://evolve.elsevier.com/cs/product/9780323653862?role=student
3. https://www.mheducation.com/highered/mhp/product/first-aid-usmle-step-1-2025.html
4. https://www.mheducation.com/highered/mhp/product/first-aid-usmle-step-2-ck-eleventh-edition.html

N. Brownstone, *The Ultimate Medical Student Guide to Dermatology*,
https://doi.org/10.1007/978-3-031-98765-6

Index

N. Brownstone, *The Ultimate Medical Student Guide to Dermatology*, https://doi.org/10.1007/978-3-031-98765-6

MIX
Papier aus verantwortungsvollen Quellen
Paper from responsible sources
FSC® C105338

If you have any concerns about our products,
you can contact us on
ProductSafety@springernature.com

In case Publisher is established outside the EU,
the EU authorized representative is:
Springer Nature Customer Service Center GmbH
Europaplatz 3, 69115 Heidelberg, Germany

Printed by Libri Plureos GmbH
in Hamburg, Germany